Older People, Nursing and Mental Health

Edited by

Stuart J. Darby
James Marr
Alan Crump
and Maria Scurfield

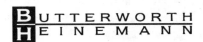

OXFORD AUCKLAND BOSTON JOHANNESBURG MELBOURNE NEW DELHI

Butterworth-Heinemann
Linacre House, Jordan Hill, Oxford OX2 8DP
225 Wildwood Avenue, Woburn, MA 01801-2041
A division of Reed Educational and Professional Publishing Ltd

 A member of the Reed Elsevier plc group

First published 1999

British Library Cataloguing in Publication Data
A catalogue record for this book is available from the British Library

ISBN 0 7506 2440 X

Typeset by Bath Typesetting
Printed and bound in Great Britain by Biddles Ltd, Guildford and King's Lynn

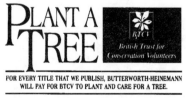

FOR EVERY TITLE THAT WE PUBLISH, BUTTERWORTH-HEINEMANN
WILL PAY FOR BTCV TO PLANT AND CARE FOR A TREE.

Contents

List of Contributors

Susan Anstey MSocSi, RMN
Sue has worked with older people for much of her fifteen years' clinical practice. Having undertaken further nursing studies in this specialist field, she conducted research into the effects of relocation on older people with mental illness as a senior student at the University of Kent at Canterbury. This work led to the successful relocation of patients when managing the development of services and standards for the Maidstone Priority Care NHS Trust. Sue continued to strive in improving services as a training manager and as the Quality Manager for the Invicta Community Care NHS Trust, helping staff to develop improved standards of practice and audit through a team approach. She also completed an MSocSi in 'Managing Quality in Health Care' at Birmingham University, and has been involved in developing staff competencies both locally and nationally.

Alan Crump BSc(Hons), RGN, RMN
Alan has worked almost exclusively with older people since he qualified from Leeds Polytechnic (now Leeds Metropolitan University) in 1986. Until recently, he was the Honorary Treasurer of the Royal College of Nursing membership group FOCUS: On Older People, Nursing and Mental Health. His previous experience has included working as a staff nurse. Alan also gained valuable experience as a support charge nurse within a King's Fund Accredited Nursing Development Unit in Leeds. He is committed to clinical practice and making every effort to break down professional, educational and social barriers to ensure that older people in distress receive the best possible care.

Stuart J. Darby MBE, BA(Hons), RGN, RMN, RHV
Stuart was originally the main editor of the book, but unfortunately died before its completion. He was Head of Community Nursing Development Team with Camden and Islington Community Health Services Trust. Stuart's employment included working as a health visitor for older people, clinical nurse specialist in mental health care of older people, and practice development nurse for community nurses working with adults and older people. He was also the chair of the Royal College of Nursing membership group FOCUS: On Older People, Nursing and Mental Health.

Niall Grant RMN, RGN

Niall Grant spent sixteen years working in a variety of areas of mental health nursing, including one year in Bellevue Hospital, New York. He later completed a PS II course in Health of Older People, continuing to develop his interest in the early onset of dementia and challenging behaviour in older men with a functional illness. Niall is presently a charge nurse at the Royal Edinburgh Hospital and is an enthusiastic user of the Nursing Development Unit Network.

Nigel Harrison BA(Hons), RGN, RMN, DPSN, PGDipEd, MA (Counselling)

Nigel is currently employed as a senior lecturer in the School of Health, Liverpool John Moore's University. His previous post was as a nurse teacher, when he facilitated pre- and postregistration courses focusing on nursing older people. Prior to teaching, Nigel was senior nurse manager (Mental Health Unit for Older People, St Charles Hospital, London) and a charge nurse in a mental health assessment ward for older people at Guy's Hospital, London.

Peter Hasler MBA, RMN

Peter Hasler is currently employed as the Director of Adult Mental Health Services for Invicta Community Care NHS Trust in Kent. He previously managed the Mental Health Services for older people in Maidstone, Kent. Peter was a founder member of the Royal College of Nursing membership group FOCUS: On Older People, Nursing and Mental Health.

Hazel Heath MSc, BA(Hons), DipN(Lond), CertEd, FETC, ITEC, RGN, RCNT, RNT

Hazel Heath is Chair of the RCN Forum for Nurses Working with Older People. As an independent nurse adviser, her work encompasses education, policy and practice development. She is also undertaking doctoral research into the nursing of older people in continuing care. Her previous posts include Senior Teacher in Nursing Theory and Practice at St Bartholomew's Hospital in London, and Adviser on Nursing and Older People to the Royal College of Nursing. Her second book *Older People and Nursing: Issues of Living in a Care Home*, edited with Pauline Ford, was short-listed by Age Concern for the 1997 Book of the Year for promoting the wellbeing and understanding of older people.

James Marr MA (Gerontology), BA (Education Studies), RGN, RMN, RCNT (DipCNE), RNT
James is currently employed as Director of Nursing at Westminster Healthcare. His previous posts have included Nurse Manager of Mental Health Services for Older People and nurse tutor specializing in nursing older people at both pre- and post-registration levels. Prior to his current post, James was a consultant nurse at Tameside Nursing Development Unit. Until recently James was the vice-chair of the Royal College of Nursing membership group FOCUS: On Older People, Nursing and Mental Health.

Liz Matthew MA, RGN, RMN
Liz Matthew trained both as a registered general and psychiatric nurse and has experience working as a community psychiatric nurse and a clinical nurse specialist, and in a variety of inpatient, day services and community clinical settings. Liz is the Directorate Manager for Services to Older People with Mental Health Problems, Tameside and Glossop Community and Priority Services NHS Trust. She has written several chapters in books relating to the care of older people with mental health problems and has just edited a book on this subject to be published later in the year.

Irene Schofield MSc (Gerontology), RGN, RNT
Irene Schofield held posts as a ward sister and senior nurse in the areas of acute admissions, assessment and rehabilitation for older people, prior to moving into nurse education, where she acted as course leader for gerontological nursing courses. She is now a locum practice nurse in East Lothian and part-time Education Fellow with The Royal College of Nursing Gerontological Nursing Programme.

Maria Scurfield BSc(Hons), RMN, DPNS
Maria is currently employed as a Practice Development Nurse in Psychiatry of Old Age at Priority Healthcare Wearside NHS Trust. Having qualified in 1984, she has worked almost exclusively with older people. Her previous experience included working as Sister of the Grange Day Unit, an assessment and treatment centre for older people with mental health needs. Prior to her current post, Maria was a Clinical Nurse Manager in Psychiatry of Old Age Directorate. Until recently Maria was the Honorary Secretary of the Royal College of Nursing membership group FOCUS: On Older People, Nursing and Mental Health.

Tracey Sharp RMN, DipHSR, MSc (Advanced Research Methods)
Tracey Sharp began her psychiatric nursing career in 1981 at Cherry Knowle Hospital, Sunderland. As a ward sister she specialized in the field of elderly care. From 1987 she worked as a research nurse, undertaking a series of research projects into the needs of carers supporting elderly people with mental health problems. She also served on the RCN FOCUS Executive Committee. In 1991, she was seconded to Sunderland Health Authority as a quality assurance officer and then later moved to Sunderland's Acute Trust where she currently works as Executive Assistant/Complaints Manager for City Hospitals Sunderland.

Foreword

When I was a student nurse one of the few placements that I really enjoyed was in mental health. There were two reasons for this. I was allowed to be me and the patients were accepted for whatever and who ever they were. The unit was well supported and led by an inspirational senior nurse who personally supervised all student nurses placed within the unit. As a result I had the opportunity to genuinely apply theory to practice, to reflect on what I experienced and I was allocated patients to work with on a one-to-one basis. I developed case study accounts to support my learning, sometimes being able to actually involve the patients in the writing of them. Such a placement was in stark contrast to my first ward experience – that of a general ward for older people.

It was during my mental health placement that I witnessed first hand 'expert nursing'. I do not know what impact this had on the patients, but for me it was a therapeutic experience – for the first time in my training I felt cared about and supported. I also had a strong sense of being valued for what I could contribute. I learnt about the importance of relationships, communication skills and the need for time. Time to spend with patients 'walking along side'. At that time I was very unaware that I had landed in an oasis of good practice greatly facilitated by adequate resources.

What is often not highlighted in studies of nursing is the systematic disadvantages which nurses and older people have had to cope with. This of course cannot excuse poor nursing practice but it does help to explain and understand it. A parallel could be drawn with an individual or family systematically disadvantaged in society by inadequate finance, substandard education, impoverished and unsuitable housing and support provided by unskilled, untrained and disinterested personnel. Traditionally, nursing has been regarded as one of the professional groups that engaged in a series of practices and behaviours which focused on ritual and control. This was the care that so many of us witnessed as student nurses in the 1970s.

Nursing older people who have mental health needs has now largely cast off the shackles of its legacy and has overcome the majority of the challenges presented by these. Through overcoming these challenges it has become one of the most pioneering, courageous and innovative areas of practice. Despite this there remains poor practice to challenge. Mental Health Nurses have had to fight for recognition of their skill and what they offer to the lives and health of older people. As a consequence there is a growing band of nurses working who have developed superb assertion skills and are very able to confront ageist, discriminatory practice in the work place. These nurses have had to be open to the realities and challenges of practice, flexible and responsive to needs and creative in finding new ways of working to develop practice and services within which they work. Many nurses feel they have to permanently fight for their client group; sometimes we forget to stop fighting and get labelled as 'difficult' and 'stroppy'.

Nurses choosing to work with older people have consistently challenged prevailing attitudes and behaviours, resulting in greater clarity about the nature of expert practice in gerontological nursing. The editors hope this book helps to clarify some of the attributes of expert nursing which take place with older people who have mental health needs – at a time when so many nurses feel that the skills, knowledge and expertise of expert nursing in the speciality are unrecognized and in danger of being lost. The expert nurse engages in holistic practice through the utilization of different sources of knowledge. In addition the nurse identifies the most pertinent issues in the situation and ways of responding to them. The nurse uses skilled judgement to determine the most appropriate response. Engagement with the patient is set within a humanistic moral framework that values the patient as a person, respecting her dignity and maintaining integrity in the situation. The expert nurse's actions are highly proficient and attuned to the situation in a way which is shaped by the patient's responses.

Those of us who work together at the RCN believe that good practice in nursing is dependent on nurses seeing their role as an enabler of health, based on individual life choices and potentials. From such a basis, outcomes from nursing can be demonstrated and our current work on the 'assessment of older people's need for nursing' clearly demonstrates this. Nurses need to be able to define and measure their contribution to the overall well-being of patients. Clearly those of us working with older people who have mental health needs know that this is often not the priority and therefore traditional, valued methods of demonstrating outcomes are denied us. As a result, nursing and patient outcomes can be hard to identify and articulate which in turn impacts on the way nursing is perceived, which leads us to consider the educational preparation of nurses for the future.

Overall there are many opportunities to influence and shape the development of mental health services for older people and clinical practice in gerontological nursing. The RCN has chosen to approach such opportunities through the development of an integrated programme of policy, development, research and education activities and we have now encapsulated all our work in a Gerontological Nursing Programme.

The importance of skilled, expert caring nursing practice can never be overestimated in the care of older people (RCN 1997). Older people should not 'suffer' because of the care they receive from nurses. Humanistic nursing tries to give the patient as many opportunities as possible to exercise freedom of choice, to express opinions, to make decisions, to talk while the nurse really listens and to have the opportunity to express their authentic self.

Given that my clinical experience of mental health was so positive I guess it was no surprise when I started at the RCN that I would love working with the committee members of the Royal College of Nursing Membership Group Focus on Older People, Nursing and Mental Health. Stuart, Jim, Alan and Maria, the editors of this book, were members of the committee during the first four years of my time with the RCN. They epitomized for me all that could and should be good about nursing. The fact that they worked with older people who had mental health needs meant that they were working in some of the worst environments with impoverished resources. They were, however, rich with skills which resulted in them delivering a much better deal for the patients with whom they worked. The chair of the committee, Stuart Darby, taught me as much in his living as he has in his death. It is rare for a week to pass without me reflecting on his leadership and humour, his clarity of thought, his decision making and his wicked, wicked sense of humour.

This book was conceived by the four editors and turned into reality by the commitment of Stuart. After Stuart died Jim took on the key coordinating role. Its publication has been delayed – I think I speak for all of us in saying that it was hard to pick up the pieces of our lives, we missed and miss Stuart so much.

Seeing the book in print is an enormous pleasure for me, bringing to light as it does the skills, knowledge and experience of expert mental health nurses working with older people. There is a national shortage of such nurses and as a result it is sometimes hard to see the differences that such expert nursing might make to the lives of older people who have mental health needs.

This book attempts to express some of the knowledge and skills in the hope that students of nursing will turn to work with older people and in particular those who have mental health needs. We need a growing band of nurses who together will ensure that nursing for older people will only get better.

It has been (and remains so) a tremendous learning opportunity to work alongside expert mental health and older people nurses. Those of us who choose to work with older people have of course many reasons for having done so, but I rather suspect that many of you reading this foreword will resonate with some of my student experiences which only served to make me determined to work with older people.

Pauline Ford
CO Director Gerontological Nursing Programme
Royal College of Nursing

Royal College of Nursing (1997). *What a Difference a Nurse Makes – a report on the benefits of expert nursing to the clinical outcomes of nursing older people*. London: RCN.

1

Exploring the myths and stereotypes of mental health in old age

Stuart J. Darby

Introduction

Old age is a part of human development and lifestyle, about which there are many myths and stereotypical views. Assumptions about the process of ageing influence society's attitudes and behaviour towards older people. These beliefs and values impact upon older persons' perception of themselves and their position within society. Ageist attitudes can lead therefore to prejudicial and discriminatory practices that affect the provision of health and social care services.

This chapter aims to explore the ways in which mental health nurses can address the stereotypes of old age. It will provide an overview of these myths and present examples of the ways in which ageism is formed and displayed. Finally, the chapter sets out to consider the approaches that nurses can take to address attitudes and behaviour that are detrimental to the wellbeing of all older people.

Ageism

The term 'ageism' was first used by Butler (1985), who linked the same bias and prejudice displayed in sexism and racism to the behaviour shown towards older people. Ageism has been defined as a set of widely shared generalizations about the characteristics of older people, which may contain an element of truth but are generally simplistic assumptions that become one-sided, exaggerated and normally prejudicial to a group of people (Abercrombie et al., 1988). Ageism can therefore lead to inequitable treatment and discrimination towards older people (Secord and Backman, 1974). As a consequence of prejudice, older people may be denied the same rights as younger people or be denied access to appropriate forms of health and social care simply because of their age and regardless of their physical and mental abilities.

Unlike sexism and racism, ageism can be generally more covert and subtle in its manifestation, with the attitudes of society shaping the social policies that govern it. Stevenson (1989) suggests that ageist attitudes are also considered to be a contributory factor to abuse and inadequate care in older age. Older people are therefore marginalized both by society and by individuals and can find themselves in a position where they are looked upon with a contempt that leads to discrimination, violation of rights and abuse, and inadequate care.

Social and demographic foundation

Social policy is often based upon demographic information in relation to age and not on epidemiological needs and trends. The provision of health and social care services may therefore be planned on the basis of, for example, the number of children under school age and the number of people over retirement age. Demographic trends over time have shown that the proportion of older people has increased over the last century, due in part to the decreases in adult mortality, infant mortality and fertility rates. In addition, these numbers are set to rise. In 1990 there were 10.5 million people over pensionable age, a rise of over one million since 1971. These numbers are expected to reach 14.5 million by the year 2031, which will be a rise of nearly forty per cent on the 1990 figures (Social Trends, 1992).

The problem with using raw data to provide a simple analysis of need is that the experience of ageing is often viewed as being the same for everyone. All people over retirement age are therefore characterized as one single homogeneous group irrespective of the diversity of their circumstances before the onset of old age. They are often portrayed as dependent, lacking in social autonomy, unloved, neglected by their immediate family, and as a burden on society, who consume without producing. In addition, older people also run the risk of being labelled 'mentally ill' when they are unable or unwilling to keep pace with present-day thinking.

Population figures can also be used to organize older people into a second negative method of division, by ranking people into 'young elderly' and 'old elderly' subgroups. This brings its own myths, with the former being considered to belong to a twilight group of grandparents who are white-haired and loving individuals, while the latter are perceived as suffering from incontinence, immobility and mental instability. Both stereotypes can, however, set out to paint the older person as a ridiculed figure, who is worthless, slow and unproductive.

Mental health in old age

To a large extent, the view of mental health in old age is based upon stereotypical views about the process of mental health changes. These myths include assumptions that old age brings about a decline in mental health that is irreversible and largely associated with 'senility', that little can be done about it, and that there is no point in early detection since there is no treatment.

As with any other age group, older people suffer from various forms of illness. The stigma of deteriorating mental health, however, is a powerful deterrent to seeking out and accepting help with mental health problems, particularly when fears of being labelled 'mad' or committed to institutional care are also present. Two major categories are used to define 'medical' mental ill health in old age. These include organic mental illness, in which definite changes in cerebral function take place, albeit for a temporary period, and functional mental disorders, where no specific physical cause can be found.

Current estimates suggest that between six and ten per cent of all older people have some degree of identifiable organic brain disturbance, namely dementia. Even in the very oldest groups, however, only a third of them experience some degree of organic brain deterioration and then usually not to such an extent that it impairs their ability to function normally in the community (Joseph, 1986).

Functional illness, including disturbances of mood, such as depression, affects about a quarter of the elderly population. It is fairly rare, however, for a clinical affective disorder to manifest itself for the first time in old age. The majority of disorders are found in older people who have a history of a similar problem in earlier life. Where the onset of an affective disorder takes place in later life, attributes such as the death of a significant person, removal from home, or some other exogenous cause, are indicated (Gearing and Slater, 1988).

In addition to this, a large proportion of mental health problems in old age can be related to temporary or permanent sensory losses, ill health and the physical effects of medicines (Stokes, 1987). A significant relationship between lifestyle events and mental health in old age can also be seen. The prominent milestone event of retirement includes altered lifestyle, altered relationships and altered personal image.

Altered lifestyle arises from the exchange of employment and paid activity for retirement and increased 'leisure time'. Although some theories promote this as a fair exchange (Dowd, 1975), the impact of reduced income, possible changes to housing, and a general disturbance of 'normal' lifestyle, are all factors that could influence an individual to such an extent that mental health problems may ensue. Altered relationships occur where partners are required to spend more time together in the home and include a number of factors such as the movement of families away from parents, the loss of work colleagues and interests, and the loss of peers and relatives through death. These are all considered to impact upon the loss and bereavement process associated with the phase of retirement. Finally, older people in retirement can develop an altered image of themselves. In addition to physical biological changes, their worth, value and status, combined with society's expectations about how they should behave or act, serve to change the way in which they perceive themselves and their role and function in the community (Palmore, 1985).

Self-concept and ideal self-concept, in which an individual tries to match up to the expectations of others or what they ought to be, have been said to create problems when individual expectations cannot be met. This leads to loss of self-esteem and loss of control which perpetuates myths, stereotypes and expectations by others.

Mental ill health in old age is therefore made up of a complex set of biological, psychological and social interactions. One of the enduring stereotypes about old age is that physical and mental illnesses are attributed to the process of ageing and therefore appropriate assessment, treatment and diagnosis are not sought. The old adage 'it's your age my dear' has been used in the past to attribute illness to ageing and could possibly be used when there are limited resources and there is a need to prioritize health and social care to those deemed to be more 'needy'. Although statistics show that the fraction of old people consulting their own general practitioner increases with age, there is some evidence that they also under-consult for their level of morbidity in comparison to younger age groups (Ford, 1985).

Given the range of factors that can contribute to mental health and well-being in old age, it can be seen that mental illness is not inevitable. Many of these factors will respond well to improved attitudes towards ageing and to nursing, medical, psychological and social care and intervention.

Sociological perspectives

Images of ageing exist at two levels: the personal image held by individuals themselves, and the images held by the wider society. It is important, therefore, to understand the way in which relative status is applied by society and the impact this has upon the self-image of older people.

Societal images and status

Although ageing is a biological process, growing older is a social process determined by the attitudes, expectations, culture and traditions of society. The theories of 'modernization' and 'idealism' can be considered as examples of the socialization process applied to ageing. Modernization theory considers that social structure can affect the altered status of older people, while idealism considers that society demands more equality between the younger population and the older population.

Modernization theory

Modernization theory focuses on the lowered status of older people and on shifts in social structures in modern industrial society). Negative stereotyping is said to be a result of transformations from a traditional agricultural society to an industrial society. This perspective provides a 'moving picture' of how society's attitudes towards older people have been shaped over a period of time.

Before modernization, the bulk of the population was located in rural areas. The levels of education and literacy were generally low and links were closely tied between extended families in which tradition was the basis of culture. After modernization, it is purported that urban environments, public education and nuclear families became the norm. Coupled with this came the evolution of the welfare state and its associated services. Innovation rather than tradition formed a new central cultural component of everyday life.

Shifts in social structures are therefore seen to be the central causal factors in modernization theory. Beliefs and values are seen as being of little importance in themselves, and behaviour is seen to reflect the dominant structure of society. The effect has been to reduce the status of older people. Examples provided by Cowgill and Holmes (1972) include:

1. Older people once derived a high status because of their rarity, since fewer people lived into old age before the improvements in health and social care.

2. Retirement (an institution in its own right) decreases the status of older people in terms of society's most valued medium of status, namely, money. Modern economic technology has created new occupations and forced out old trades, so that experience is a less valued position.

3. Greater geographical mobility and urbanization has been said to have destroyed extended family networks and destroyed the status of older people who were often a necessary source of financial and social support systems.
4. Finally, public mass education has led to widespread literacy and has challenged the position of older people as transmitters of cultural knowledge and wisdom.

Idealist theory

Idealism offers an alternative to modernization theory. Fischer (1978) considers that political and social revolutions have changed the order of respect, deference and reverence afforded to older people. As a result of these conflicts, society demands more equality between the younger and older populations.

In this sense, idealism emphasizes a shift from social structural arrangements (modernization) causing a breakdown in relationships between young and old, to factors relating to the experience of ageing. Individual knowledge and experience of the external world therefore influences the way in which we interpret and define it (Gross, 1987). Examples of the ways in which shifts in relationships between younger and older people can affect status include:

1. The past admiration for the wisdom and experience of older people has disappeared, for example, where skills and trades needed to be taught and passed down between generations because of a demand for equality by younger people (Palmore, 1985).
2. Older people have been eased out of key positions in situations where there has been a growth in technology, political advancement and a 'cult of youth'.
3. A breakdown in social institutions, such as close family networks and reliance upon support from older relatives, has led to less value being placed on the importance of the role of older people (O'Donnell, 1981).

Status within industrial societies therefore changes with retirement. Legislation dictates that older persons become old as a consequence of retirement and not on the basis of their physical or mental abilities. In preindustrial society, older people often had greater status since their knowledge, wisdom and contribution to everyday living was based upon their life experience and not their ability to earn money or work productively.

Preparation for old age and expectations for the future have been said, therefore, to be derived from long-term social changes. Lasch (1980) considers that these changes occur through attitudes that have at their roots an irrational fear, panic and terror of old age and death, and that these attitudes are associated with narcissistic personalities as the dominant type of personality structure in contemporary society. Individuals look to others to compare and validate their sense of themselves. The inability of older persons to be admired for beauty, charm or power leads to their inability to achieve through work or love. Self-destruction takes place, as older people become unable to live vicariously through their children; eventually, this leads to further 'fraying' of links between generations.

Psychological perspectives

Individual attitudes, values and beliefs about the process of ageing are influenced, therefore, by what a person believes objectively, what a person feels subjectively and the behaviour or way in which a person responds to these feelings and values. Although growing up is normally taken to be something desirable and almost an end in itself, growing old has traditionally had very negative connotations.

Self-image and status

Contrasting psychological theories provide illustrations of the way in which self-image of ageing can affect the individual older person. Examples of these psychological theories include 'the decrement model', 'social exchange theory' and the 'disengagement theory'.

The decrement model is a term used to describe a negative image of ageing (Gross, 1987). The fundamental characteristics include decay or decline in physical and mental health and a reduction in intellect and social relationships. In contrast, the social exchange theory stresses the potential and advantages of increased leisure time and a reduction in day-to-day responsibilities. Dowd (1974) suggests that older people give up paid employment to receive honourable discharge and increased leisure time. This is seen as a 'contract for older people'. Although individuals may want to refuse to undertake this contract, societal expectations and social pressure can often force them to withdraw from society. This image is clearly a conflict of interest affecting individuals and over which they have little or no control.

Finally, the disengagement theory concentrates on the way in which older people withdraw from society. Cumming and Henry (1961) consider that work and social life are inextricably linked. When retirement takes place, this link is broken, resulting in disengagement from the society and world that these older people once knew. Disengagement theory attempts to explain why people play a less important role in old age than they do in middle age. It holds that retiring from important social roles performs important functions both for society as a whole and for the individual older members of society. Freedom from the burden and responsibility of work and the conservation of energy to perform tasks found to be meaningful are proposed benefits. The theory itself, however, has been attacked as promoting negative images, although most people do express a wish to give up paid employment and to retire from full-time occupation (Havighurst, 1963).

This perspective, therefore, views society as being composed of competing and conflicting groups, rich versus poor and young versus old (Morris and Williamson, 1982). The issue of retirement from paid occupation has clear disadvantages in loss of status, decreased income and reduced societal value in the eyes of society. The amount of control that a person feels that they have over their life style and future is clearly linked to them succumbing to ageist policies that impact upon their feelings of self-worth and value.

Research

Although there is some agreement on the biological changes occurring in ageing, there is little research-based agreement on the psychological dimensions. As with physical status, the popular image of psychological health in old age is one of gradual but inevitable decline.

There have been research attempts to provide a scientific and true picture of 'normal' mental health changes in old age. Of the three types of methodology commonly used to investigate these changes, namely cross-sectional, longitudinal and sequential studies, each has problems in avoiding the bias associated with stereotyping (Ford, 1985). Many of the studies by which pessimistic conclusions are reached are based upon research that reflects the inferences attributed to ageing.

Cross-sectional studies compare age differences between age groups. They do not therefore reveal individual age changes. This can lead to overgeneralizations about groups of people which are consequently applied to all older people.

Longitudinal studies compare people over a given period of time. Inevitably, some may die during this period, leaving perhaps the fittest and intellectually most able at the end of the study. This serves to present a skewed picture that is not truly representative of the total number of people under investigation.

Sequential studies have problems in removing all the variables that have been mentioned earlier. These variables may include environment, culture and ageist attitudes. Studies have shown that variables such as life style development and differences between people born as little as ten years apart, living in rural or industrial areas, and having different education, nutrition, medical care and employment opportunities, can all contribute to intellectual and mental health development (Gearing and Slater., 1988).

The difficulty with research studies is that, while attempting to provide a snapshot of the reality of mental health in old age that can be generalized to a larger group of people, they cannot always reflect or provide answers to meeting individual needs. Building upon personal abilities, using the past history and background of older people, can be crucial to planning care services and meeting individual care needs.

The major areas of psychological investigation and research include the decline of learning abilities, memory, personality changes and intelligence. All are considered to be prominent features of mental health changes in old age.

Learning and memory

Learning is related to the ability to perform a task and commit this performance to memory in order for the same task to be carried out on a future occasion in the same or a similar way. Data relating to memory and learning in work situations show that, given a longer training period, many older people do manage to learn, but that the degree of success is likely to depend upon the nature of the task, its relationship to previous experience, and the method of training (Chown, 1981). Expectations by the rest of society therefore pose a major problem in the learning ability of older people. Anxiety in new learning situations and the time taken to complete tasks completely and competently, for example payment at supermarket checkouts, leads to a societal expectation of incompetence. The problem therefore lies not in the ability to continue to function intellectually, but in the lack of opportunity and time to process information in the learning period.

Memory problems may be a feature of old age, particularly where a diagnosis of dementia has been made. It is unlikely, however, for a younger person to be considered to have a mental health problem if they inadvertently leave a tap running or forget to lock the front door, as it would be for an older person.

Personality traits

The personality traits of older people often arouse negative views and can be seen in the language used to describe their personality. 'Withdrawn', 'isolated' and 'emotionally unstable' are descriptive words found in common usage. Personality surveys conducted by Age Concern (1974) showed that older people do not feel that they change as they age, and that they still possess the same traits, attributes and characteristics. However, if the opportunities for social activities are reduced, then an individual may deal with this by becoming more introverted and withdrawn. The response of an older person could therefore be seen as an internal reaction rather than as a process of ageing. What is 'normal' and what is desirable are clearly key factors in differentiating between personality change occurring as a result of old age and personality change as a way of dealing with the situation in which older people find themselves.

Many of the studies on intelligence testing in older people and the identification of age differences in intellectual function are based upon cross-sectional studies. Decreased intellectual performance with age, therefore, may well just reflect differences in the educational levels of cohorts. It could also be argued that intelligence itself does not change with age but that skills and information held by older people become obsolete. Changes in technology, new equipment and advanced methods of working, for example, the computerization and automation of equipment, tend to be anathema to people who are unfamiliar with these systems.

In psychological tests, older people seem to sacrifice speed for accuracy, perhaps reflecting their general feelings of inadequacy. When time limits are removed from psychological experiments, age differences in performance are much less marked and older people achieve and perform tasks that measure learning in a manner that is equal to younger subjects (Chown, 1981).

Current research-based evidence shows that ageing does not bring about an inevitable and profound decline in mental ability (Gearing and Slater 1988). Older people can learn and improve their intellectual functioning, given the right sort of educational programmes and the right setting. The increasing popularity of the University of the Third Age in a variety of countries testifies to the general high level of intellectual functioning and desire for education amongst older people (University of the Third Age, 1984). Older people learn best in nonthreatening environments in which they regain confidence in their own abilities. The scope for reteaching skills when physical or mental illness has reduced an individual's functional ability clearly needs to be taken into account. However, as with physiological changes, it is difficult to distinguish between what is due to ageing alone and what part cultural and environmental factors play.

Examples of ageism

Chronological ageing

Chronological ageing myths relate to the way in which all older people are considered to belong to one homogeneous group, sharing the same values and the same life style, and therefore acting and behaving within a given range of functions. The physical 'look' and mental abilities of persons are simply related therefore to the number of years that they have lived. Although it is true that older people are more likely to experience ill health and disability in later years, it is not necessarily an inevitable consequence of the ageing process.

This view, however, can be easily reinforced, since health professionals usually come into contact with a disproportionate number of older people and this serves to augment their views and attitudes. The consequent danger is that health and social care providers will either undertreat or overprovide. On the one hand is a tendency to deny older people access to the most up-to-date or more expensive treatments, while on the other there is overprovision of care that reduces independence and freedom of rights. In this way chronological age definitions serve to reinforce views of increasing dependence upon others.

Rejection and isolation

Loneliness is a trait that is often attributed to older people. In reality, only about 20 per cent of people over 65 years of age live entirely alone and assumptions must be made that some actually do this out of choice. Joseph (1986) considers that those people who live in residential or nursing home accommodation are more likely to be childless, the poorest in financial and social terms, and without siblings.

It is frequently said that children find their ageing parents sickly and boring, and edge them out of the family. Although it is clear that changes in the size of families and the participation of women in the labour market over the past century will have a marked effect on the number and availability of family members to provide care for older dependents in their own homes, there are, however, few data to support the view that the families neglect the care of those who are old and dependent when services are provided by the state. Older people are also able to contribute to family life by taking responsibilities within the home as well as contributing financially through independent income and pensions. The flow of help and assistance is not therefore unidirectional and demonstrates that reciprocal care arrangements do take place within families.

The unquestioning acceptance of rejection may serve to reinforce government policy of putting pressure upon carers, relatives and neighbours to provide care in the community instead of looking at strategies for meeting health and social care needs based upon the number of people over a certain age, their individual abilities, housing stock and financial income.

Self-fulfilling prophecies

Individual images of ageing and self-concept are based upon the attributes that people ascribe to themselves, and which can also be linked to societal and cultural expectations. Self-concept, beliefs and behaviour of older people have been shown to be the result of ageist attitudes. Older people are more inclined to behave in a way in which society expects them to do. They therefore collude with a social construction of reality and see themselves as a group apart (French, 1990). The impact of this may be that people delay in seeking medical and social help, since they attribute problems to ageing and do not wish to present themselves as a burden to health and social care providers, or indeed to family and friends (Haug 1986). Clearly, this can then exacerbate problems and contribute further to negativistic attitudes. Older people fail to seek financial benefits and opportunities because this serves to reinforce their feelings of inadequacy and unworthiness, and of having charitable status that takes without giving in return. The resulting behaviour of older people has therefore been said to be in alignment with societal expectations and not with the expectations of the older people themselves (Midwinter, 1986).

It is not the young alone who have negative expectations of old age (Gearing and Slater 1988). Gerontophobia (the fear of ageing) is present in many people until they become 'old' themselves. By recognizing that life is not so terrible for them, they then consider themselves to be exceptions to the rule and thus add to the stereotypes and myths of old age. Problems that affect some older people (often a minority) are then presented by an 'overdrawn' picture of an inevitable decline that is seen as a necessary accompaniment of old age and entrenching an 'inevitable myth' (Saul, 1974). In the long term, images that are often intended to generate concern about the real and serious problems of some older people can actually perpetuate a negative effect.

Gender and sexuality

Discussions about old age are often largely concentrated on women. There are twice as many women as men who are aged sixty-five years and four times as many at seventy-five years. Older women experience both ageism and sexism, being discriminated against because they are both old and female. Thomas (1988) considers that this double disadvantage is both socially defined and socially constructed.

The attributes of male masculinity are associated with qualities such as competence, autonomy and self-control, and are combined with stereotypes such as 'grey hair in males is distinguishing' and 'older men make better lovers'. This serves to denigrate even further the qualities for which women are commonly desired: beauty, physical attractiveness and child bearing. The feminist movement has been criticized for contributing to this gender issue through concentrating on the issues raised by young women, such as abortion, contraception and premenstrual syndromes, and ignoring the needs of older women (Macdonald, 1984).

Older women are also handicapped because they can no longer fulfil a reproductive function and are considered to be less sexually attractive. It is commonplace to consider that sexuality is not a prerequisite in old age and that older people have little exploitable value for both the contraception and pornography industries (Andrews, 1989). An example of this surrounds the beliefs about the risk factors associated with HIV and AIDS. Surveys have shown that universal precautions are rarely taken with older people. It is considered that people aged over sixty-five years were, generally speaking, raised in an era when sexual morality was much more conservative and are therefore not likely to be sexually active in old age (Sadler, 1993). Recent reports have indicated the danger of assuming that HIV and AIDS is a younger person's problem. 'A crisis in silence' (Age Concern, 1993) considers that the number of older people with HIV is likely to be underestimated, simply because of ageist attitudes about older people and their sexual life styles.

This difference in outlook provides further evidence to support the views that older people are repressed and unexciting. Society is therefore much more permissive about ageing in men, giving older single men greater status than unmarried women, sanctioning men marrying women many years their junior and yet considering it to be humorous when older women have younger male partners. There is also evidence to suggest that males who are disabled and living at home, or are providing care for a female dependent, are more likely to receive support at home, such as meals on wheels and home help, than women in the same situation (Charlesworth et al., 1984). Phillipson (1982) suggests that because the majority of older people in institutional care are women, the standards may be lower and that women were far more likely than men to be depersonalized on admission to a geriatric ward (Evers, 1981).

In this context, D'A Slevin (1991) conducted a study of the attitudes of student and newly qualified nurses. The results demonstrated not only a rise in negative attitudes in nurses during their period of training but also that males demonstrated more negative attitudes than their female counterparts.

Ethnicity

In addition to the double-edged sword of ageism and sexism is the vulnerability of being old and black (Curtis, 1991). Although one in five people over the age of sixty-five years is white, only one in twenty belong to black and ethnic minority groups (Social Trends, 1992).

Skodra (1991) found that in psychological assessments of older black women, the content, process and outcome of psychological testing was affected by the ethnicity of the women being investigated. First, there was little reference made in relation to information gathering about the background culture of these people, how this experience had affected their lives and whether they were able to achieve their expectations and personal goals. Secondly, the beliefs of the health professionals themselves were considered to be at fault, since they had a tendency to regard everything as having a psychosocial pathology. Thirdly, there was the important issue of validating the older black women's experiences, concerns, fears and feelings. Culturally biased testing, for example asking for the date of the First World War, when this may not have a been part of their past life experience or a significant life event, served to work against older persons and relegated them to lower cognitive scores.

Sollit and Hornsey (1990) consider that the status of being 'elderly' must be resumed in the same way that 'black' has been reclaimed as a positive affirmation of the cultural identity, wealth of experience, and values and beliefs of black and ethnic minority individuals.

Media images

The images that society holds of old age are represented and reflected in the various aspects of popular culture and mass media. The presentation of materials relating to older people, including nonverbal aspects, tends to relate to a certain level of emotional appeal. This could be said to be one of the most important ways in which society transmits social norms and expectations. The message, through television, radio, printed matter, advertisements and public entertainment, can be a blatant form of ageism.

Although a culture of youth is used to advertise and promote health, beauty and leisure activity products, older people are used to promote laxatives, pain formulas and dental adhesives. Advertisements and popular journals present the ultimate image and achievements of younger 'beautiful people' by sexual imagery that is seen to be playing a major part in influencing our life style.

On the whole, older people (with the exception of politicians) are conspicuous by their absence on television or in the mass media. When they appear in fictional works, they are generally portrayed as background characters, mostly of middle class status. Reasonable health and fitness is depicted amongst the young elderly, although sexuality and dominance are played down. Senility, neglect and abuse is the focus of attention in older elderly people and is mostly directed towards women. Covert forms of ageism exist in day-to-day examples showing older people being different and outstanding if they have achieved athletic feats.

Heath (1989) cites covert 'ageism by apartheid', in the form of shops that offer 'reduced rates' (but only on specified days) and birthday cards that strengthen, reinforce and maintain ageist views on growing older, rather than a celebration of life. Heath considers that this subtle form of ageism would not be tolerated by other groups in society who are also the targets of negative stereotyping. There would be a major outcry against statements such as: 'People with learning disabilities told to live in one room – to keep warm' and 'Gays and Blacks half price – Mondays only'.

Professional images

Norman (1987) believes that gerontology tends to take a 'victim blaming' approach, looking for problems with older persons themselves rather than looking for a much wider societal cause. She cites the example of hypothermia, which is put down to age rather than to the fact that low income and poor housing conditions are more likely to contribute to this condition. It has been these changes that have prompted the perception of older people as a 'social problem'.

Attitudes among professionals

In addition to the economics and rationing of health care in old age, individual attitudes of professionals themselves can lead to further ageist treatment. D'A Slevin (1991) reports the results of a study using an inventory designed to investigate the attitudes of young adults. The study set out to investigate and consider the implications for a caring profession, since it is suggested that older people will represent the most common care group for nursing in the future. The study found that the attitudes of student nurses changed for the worse on becoming newly qualified. A number of factors were thought to contribute to this outcome, including the omission of older adults as a specialist area in the Project 2000 educational structure for nurses. 'Doctrinal conversion' was also thought to be one of the contributing factors. This concerns the internalization of a body of professional attitudes and behaviour because of a disease-orientated approach to care provision that values high technology and devalues less acute care. The findings supported the fact that professional socialization, including education, led to nurses having institutionalized and negative attitudes towards older people as a part of their professional cultural beliefs.

Working status

Working with older people has always assumed low status in the past, while working with older people with mental health needs has also perhaps been the Cinderella of all Cinderella services. A number of health professionals are still shown to believe that older people are the least deserving when resources and services are being distributed (Wetle, 1987). The prestige associated with acute medical care and 'life saving' techniques is not apparent when older people are receiving care. Norman (1987) considers that this has in the past been a factor in attracting less skilled workers, who are usually people who are subject to discrimination themselves. Skill mix and changes in the ratios of qualified to unqualified staff is a development that has recently been under discussion. The provision of care for older people has been one of the main target areas in which a 'cheaper' option of providing unqualified staff is considered in an attempt to maximize on limited resources. Under-resourcing and the low status and kudos associated with working with older people with mental health needs has therefore contributed to the past problems of providing adequate and appropriate services. Although this group of people are in the age group most at risk, they are the one group that health and social care services have been least likely to serve (Charny and Lewis, 1986).

Professional language

In addition to low status and underresourcing, many of our attitudes are shaped and reflected in the language used by professionals. Nurses have been cited as using terms of endearment such as 'gran', 'old love' or first name terms that serve to embarrass and patronize older people. Day (1988) considers that this is putting the person in a childlike role: submissive, vulnerable, in need of protection and dependent. This also suggests power over a person, with the balance towards the professional who is using such terminology without first seeking permission or asking that person how they would prefer to be addressed. Although there has been a general shift away from the use of 'geriatric' as a noun, terms such as 'elderly' and 'aged' can also give the impression that all older people belong to one homogeneous group. 'Care of the elderly' would also not be acceptable if it were applied to 'care of the young' or 'care of the middle aged', since this conjures up a dependent state rather than promoting independence and self-fulfilment.

Health economics

Stammers (1992) considers the expense of providing medical care for older people. In general practitioner prescribing alone, older people are responsible for forty-one per cent of prescriptions, while some eighty-seven per cent of those aged over sixty-five years are taking regular medication and a third will be taking more than three drugs.

Whitaker (1991) describes how the principles of health economics are inherently ageist if used to choose between the provision of care between patients of different ages. He considers that the National Health Service is already biased towards ageist social and demographic trends and that the current reforms in progress will provide much potential for discrimination. Choices and rationing over what services will be offered to patients will become more necessary and more difficult.

Health economics is about making rational choices in order to make the 'best' use of available resources. There are, however, many different kinds of rationality. In order to make rational choices between different ways of spending resources, health economists must compare activities in terms of the costs and the benefits.

Whitaker describes the 'social' model of health economics, which advocates that everyone is worthy of treatment and attention. If resources are to be limited, they should be limited across the board. Conversely, under an 'economic' model, if resources are to be limited they should be selective in order to maximize the benefit per unit cost. A proportion of the funding therefore is allocated and dictated by the perceived worth of the person receiving it.

When these models are applied using a method such as 'quality adjusted life years', two markers are used to estimate the cost and the benefit (Harris, 1987). These are the number of years of life gained as a result of treatment or intervention, and the quality of those years. It is easy to see that, when a scientific value is used to weight a scoring system, younger people are more likely to score highly and therefore be perceived as benefiting the most from any treatment or care.

Day (1988) suggests as an exercise in challenging professional ageism that we should conduct assessments or planning exercises without referring to a person's age. The activity of describing the care needs of two people without reference to age can result, therefore, in two entirely different sets of outcomes.

In systems where cost containment predominates over cost effectiveness, it is easy to see the potential for hidden discrimination against a politically inert group of people who could be hoodwinked into receiving cheaper substandard services. In addition to this, even charitable funding for services for older people is more likely to be reduced, since they do not attract the same public sympathy as, for example, services for children. Age is therefore a common factor in deciding on subsequent treatment or the way in which a person's care will be planned, offered or managed.

The nursing contribution

Nurses need to ensure that their own practice, and that of health and social service colleagues, is not founded on stereotypical views of ageing. The main areas to be discussed here include a knowledge of the ageing process and the ability to assess and identify individual needs. Insight, awareness and education into attitudes and guarding against ageist practice are also considered.

Knowledge of the ageing process

Factual evidence on the biological, social and psychological processes in relation to ageing are an important foundation for distinguishing between what is 'normal' and what constitutes myths of the ageing process. Nurses need education and training in order for them to be aware of these various aspects of ageing and to ensure that assumptions about the physical or mental abilities of a person are not attributed simply to an inevitable consequence of the ageing process.

Nurses need to have knowledge and understanding of the ways in which external influences and past life events will have shaped older people's response to their current situation. Making sense of what is happening now to individuals is dependent upon understanding what has influenced them or occurred before. Examples of these influences include cultural and historical perspectives, social order, politics, fashion and custom, and education and employment history.

In addition, there are many unique internal biographical factors that affect older people. Examples of these will include the way in which people feel about their past lifetime experiences, how their life has developed and been adjusted, and the values and expectations that they have about the present and the future. Finally, a knowledge and understanding of the way in which individuals have prepared for retirement, and the types of 'coping mechanisms' that they may have adopted, are often the keys to understanding their individual position and behaviour.

Assessment and identification of individual needs

Nurses play a vital role in assessing and identifying the mental health changes occurring in older age that may prevent older people from achieving optimum fulfilment of their lives. They can act as a central pivot between different agencies, educating, coordinating, liaising and referring to health and social care services as appropriate. Assessment provides the opportunity to plan future care needs and can be undertaken on an individual basis or with groups of people sharing the same or similar problems. Assessment therefore needs to be part of a systematic process of collecting information about older individuals and the world in which they live. It is not just about diagnosis, because it provides a baseline for further investigation and for planning to meet the current and future needs that will maintain or enhance a healthy life style.

The care programme approach (Department of Health, 1990a) and community living assessments under the NHS and Community Care Act (Department of Health, 1990b) both provide a framework for allowing older persons to access services. They also provide the opportunity for a nursing contribution to assessment to take place and for nurses to operate as part of a team offering a range of therapies and treatments and practical information. Through advocating on behalf of older people, they can ensure that they have an equitable contribution to any decision-making process, providing them with the opportunity to define their own needs and to anticipate and prevent future problems from being exacerbated or from reaching crisis point.

Insight, awareness and education

Nurses have a responsibility to address both professional and societal attitudes. Through the identification of their own personal needs in tandem with the needs of clients and patients, they can set examples to ensure that society starts to uphold different values and beliefs. The power of health professionals still influences the thoughts of many people. The provision of an appropriate, nonageist role model can do much to negate and change the attitudes of other members of society and of other professionals.

By developing insight and awareness into ageism, nurses can avoid the prejudgement of people, this environment, or the situation in which they are placed. This provides a basis for developing sensitivity, and understanding the context of the past life experiences to which people relate their current life style. Insight and awareness can also ensure that attention is paid to the use of appropriate and acceptable language that is not patronizing or belittling, but facilitates a more egalitarian power base between nurses as providers and older persons as consumers. Awareness training therefore needs to include the opportunity for exploring equality of rights, the use of risk and restraint, and, above all, ensuring that disability is not considered to be normal but is the loss of an ability that requires thorough investigation.

Those responsible for staff education, training and professional development need to consider the attitudes, values and convictions of care providers themselves. The aim should be to make the experience of ageing meaningful to health professionals and to the place in which they work. In addition, the overall outcome should assist them to identify what they believe, what they think should happen, and how their practice can be changed to reflect effective, acceptable care. Buckwalter et al. (1993) consider the use of numerous types of individual and group work exercises that use a questionnaire to identify ageist attitudes and provide targets for addressing them.

It has been shown that older people can be changed by altering the environment in which they live. They are not impervious to situational change and may respond to their own dissatisfactions with reality (Carp, 1967). When health professionals are actively involved with older people they develop more realistic and optimistic attitudes to this age group. A nonageist outlook is therefore fostered in situations where exposure to older people in society takes place. The true integration of older people into society, both in employment and as valued members in all walks of life, may promote positive imagery and negate negative preconceptions.

Guarding against ageist practice

Working within multidisciplinary teams provides nurses with the opportunity to check ageist practice. Negotiating aims and objectives for health care with both older individuals and their lay carers can help the understanding of these people's personal position and guard against making decisions in which they are not involved or which are contrary to their own wishes. Summarizing and confirming that the nurses' understanding matches that of the individuals concerned can prevent misunderstanding and actions that may be based upon stereotypical views of the abilities of older persons. The devolvment of power and responsibility, and the empowering of older people helps to ensure that they have control over their health care and that care is carried out *with* people and not *for* people.

Self-care may well be an essential strategy necessary to older people in maintaining their health. It is therefore important that they are able to operate from a position of knowledge, have the opportunity to discuss health issues, including personal relationships, and can actively participate in health education and health groups as a basic human right. Examples of this include anticipatory work and preretirement counselling. Preparation for the effects of retirement can have a major benefit and impact upon older people (Drennan, 1988).

Systematic monitoring of the way in which care is communicated and offered is therefore an essential component of providing appropriate care and empowering older people. Nursing care needs to be flexible and responsive. It must avoid prejudgement and accept individuals regardless of the environment or situation, because decisions made on behalf of older people can set up tensions that lead to non-compliance, inappropriate self-treatment and poor relationships with health professionals and lay carers (Day, 1988).

Finally, focusing on strengths rather than weaknesses is an important factor in negating self-fulfilling prophecies, guarding against ageist practice, and enabling older people to contribute to their own health and welfare. Identifying and promoting individual strengths and abilities minimize the effect of societal attitudes and assist older people to understand and differentiate between age changes and ill health in old age.

Conclusion

Ageism, based upon stereotypical views and myths about the process of ageing, leads to inequitable treatment and discrimination against older people. The problem with using data that are based simply upon numbers of older people to plan health and social care services is that the experience of ageing is then often viewed as being the same for everyone. Mental health in old age is made up of a complex set of biological, psychological and social interactions. One of the enduring stereotypes of old age is that physical and mental illnesses are attributed to the process of ageing and therefore appropriate assessment, treatment and diagnosis are not sought.

Preparation for old age and expectations for the future have been said to be derived from long-term social changes. These changes occur because of an attitude that has at its roots an irrational fear, panic and terror of old age and death. Individuals look to others to compare and validate their sense of themselves. Individual attitudes, values and beliefs about the process of ageing become influenced therefore by what a person believes objectively, what a person feels subjectively, and the way in which a person responds to these feelings and values. Although growing up is normally taken to be something desirable and almost an end in itself, growing old has traditionally built up very negative connotations.

Current research-based evidence demonstrates that ageing does not bring about an inevitable and profound decline in mental ability. Older people can learn and improve their intellectual functioning, given the right amount of time, suitable educational programmes and the right setting.

The myths of ageing are therefore compounded by societal expectations and the value and worth perceived by older people themselves. These are perpetuated by professional images and attitudes.

Fears about state expenditure on elderly people are essentially ideological views that are not always supported by biological or psychological facts. Discrimination and prejudice show society displaying an ageist attitude that demonstrates a marked a lack of concern about its older members as sexism does about women and racism does about black and ethnic minority individuals. In the long term, future generations of younger people will lose out as they change from being observers to fully participating members of an older society. The main goal for nurses therefore must be to replace notions of dependency and to foster a framework that places emphasis on interdependence between generations.

References

Abercrombie, N., Hill, S. and Turner, B. (1988). *Dictionary of Sociology.* Harmondsworth: Penguin.

Age Concern. (1974). *The Attitudes of the Elderly and Retired.* Mitcham: Age Concern.

Age Concern. (1993). *A Crisis of Silence: HIV, AIDS and Older People.* (A Resource Pack for Age Concern). London.

Andrews, J. (1989). Anti-ageists unite. *Nurs. Times Nurs. Mirror,* (85) 22.

Buckwalter, K., Smith, M. and Martin, M. (1993). Attitude problem. *Nurs. Times,* **89**(5), 55–57

Butler, R. (1985). *Why Survive? Being Old In America.* New York: Harper & Row.

Carp, F. (1967). The impact of environment on old people. *Gerontologist,* **7**, 106–108, 135.

Charlesworth, et al. (1984). *Carers and Services: a Comparison of Men and Women Caring for Dependent Elderly People.* Manchester Equal Opportunities Commission.

Charney, M. and Lewis, P. (1989). Choosing who shall not be treated in the NHS. *Soc. Sci. Med.,* **28**, 1331–1338.

Chown, S. ed. (1981). *Human Ageing: Selected Readings.* p11. Harmondsworth: Penguin.

Cowgill, D. and Holmes, L. (1972). *Aging and modernization,* 3rd ed. Cited in *In the Eye of the Beholder: Contemporary Issues in Stereotyping.* (A. Miller, ed.) pp. 69–73, New York: Praeger.

Cumming, E. and Henry, W. (1961). *Growing Old, the Process of Disengagement..* Basic Books: New York.

Curtis, Z. (1991). Redressing the balance. *Crit. Public Health,* **2**, 29–30.

D'A Slevin, O. (1991). Ageist attitudes among young adults: implications for a caring profession. *J. Adv. Nurs.,* **16**, 1197–1205.

Day, L. (1988). How ageism impoverishes elderly care, and how to combat it. *Geriatr. Med.,* **18**(2), 14–15.

Department of Health. (1990a). *The care programme approach for people with mental illness referred to the specialist psychiatric services.* (HC[90]23/LASSL[90]11.) London: DoH.

Department of Health. (1990b). The NHS and community care act. London: HMSO.

Dowd, J. (1975). Social exchange theory. In (1984). *A First Course in Psychology.* (N. Hayes) p. 317, Edinburgh: Nelson.

Drennan, V. (1988). *Health Visitors and Groups.* Oxford: Heinemann.

Evers, H. (1981). Care or Custody? *In: Controlling Women.* (B. Hutter and G. Williams, eds.) pp 61–83, London: Croom Helm.

Fischer, D. (1978). *Growing Old in America,* New York: Oxford University Press.

Ford, G. (1985). Illness behaviour in old age. In (1988) *Self Care and Health in Old Age.* K. Dean, T. Hickey and B. Holstein, pp. 130–166, London: Croom Helm.

French, S. (1990). Ageism. *Physiotherapy,* **96**, 178–181.

Gearing, B. and Slater, R. (1988). Attitudes, stereotypes and prejudice about aging. In *Mental Health Problems in Old Age,* (B. Gearing, M. Johnson and T. Heller, eds) p. 27, Milton Keynes: Open University.

Gross, R. (1987). *Psychology: the Science of Mind and Behaviour.* p. 601.

Harris, J. (1987). QALYfying the value of life. *J. Med. Ethics,* **13**, 117–123.

Haug, M. (1986). Doctor–patient relationships and their impact on elderly care. In (1988). *Self Care and Health in Old Age.* (K. Dean, T. Hickey and B. Holstein). London: Croom Helm.

Havighurst, R. (1964). Successful Ageing. In (1984). *A First Course in Psychology.* (N.

Hayes) p. 317, Edinburgh: Nelson.

Heath, H. (1989). Old: almost a four letter word? *Nurs. Times*, **85**(31), 36–37.

Joseph, J. (1986). *Sociology for Everyone*. Cambridge: Polity Press.

Lasch, C. (1980). *The Culture of Narcissism*. New York: Abacus Press. Cited in (1981). *A New Introduction to Sociology*. (M. O'Donnell). p. 387, Edinburgh: Nelson.

Macdonald, B. (1984). *Look Me in the Eye Old Woman*. London: The Women's Press.

Midwinter, E. (1986). *A Time for Age*. (Fact Pack.) London: BBC Radio 4.

Morris, M. and Williamson, J. (1982). Stereotypes and social class: a focus on poverty. In: *In the Eye of the Beholder: Contemporary Issues in Stereotyping*. (A. Miller, ed.) pp. 400–405, New York: Praeger.

Norman, A. (1987). *Aspects of Ageism: A Discussion Paper*. London: Centre for Policy on Ageing.

O'Donnell, M. (1981). *A New Introduction to Sociology*. Edinburgh: Nelson.

Palmore, E. (1985). *Retirement: Causes and Consequences*. New York: Springer.

Phillipson, C. (1982). *Capitalism and the Construction of Old Age*. London: Methuen.

Sadler, C. (1993). Positively older. *Nurs. Times*, **89**(26), 22–23.

Saul, S. (1974). *Aging: an Album of People Growing Old*. New York: John Wiley.

Skodra, E. (1991). Ageism and psychological testing with elderly immigrant women. *Counselling Psychol. Q.*, **4**, 59–63.

Social Trends. (1992). *General Statistical Services* No. 22. London: HMSO.

Sollit, L. and Hornsey, J. (1990). Tackling ageism. *J. Distr. Nurs.*, **9**(1), 22–23.

Stammers, T. (1992). What is at the root of ageism? *Care Elderly*, **4**, 288–289.

Stevenson, O. (1989). *Age and Vulnerability*. London: Edward Arnold.

Stokes, G. (1987). Self care skills and reducing institutionalised behaviour in a long-stay psychiatric population. *J. Adv. Nurs.*, **12**, 35–48.

Thomas, L. (1988). A double-edged sword. *Geriatr. Nurs. Home Care*, **8**(7), 21.

University of the Third Age. (1984). *The Image of the Elderly On Television*. (Research Report number 1.) Cambridge: University of the Third Age.

Wetle, T. (1987). Age as a risk factor for inadequate treatment. *JAMA*, **258**, 516.

Whitaker, P. (1991). The inherent ageism of health economics. *Geriatr. Med.*, **11**, 57–58.

2

*The social construction of old age and its impact on
mental health*

Liz Matthew

Introduction

The aim of this chapter is to suggest how health care professionals can improve the quality of care by understanding the social background of older people with mental health problems. It briefly covers the major theories of ageing as well as providing practical suggestions for self-development, and also examines the mental health of older people in a social context, and recognizes that the caring professions are members of a wider society and that they live within a social context of their own family, community and workplace. Taking this into account, the chapter also considers how the particular concepts of old age and mental health influence health care workers.

In the past, political and economic factors have influenced the way in which we now live and perceive others within our society. For this reason, consideration is given to both demography and theories of ageing, and how they in turn reflect or influence the thinking of the time. Particular emphasis will be placed on life style and gender.

As well as identifying the common mental health problems of old age, there is a need to put this understanding into both social and medical contexts that recognize the importance of environmental factors, as well as organic factors, on health.

The process of 'growing old' has a number of effects on an individual. The most obvious are the physical changes, such as greying of the hair, wrinkling of the skin and the slowing down of reactions to stimuli. When considering mental ill health we can add other behavioural aspects, such as those resulting from organic brain disease, but this is a very small part of the complex process of ageing. As we do not live in isolation, a key aspect of human behaviour is socialization. People function only by relating to others and have

developed complex social systems ranging from their own family relationships to being part of an international community.

The sociological context

As nurses, we commonly ignore the fact that the old woman in front of us,
who is confined to residential care and receiving no visitors, is actually part
of a more complex society. On a superficial level most of us see a physically
old and frail individual who communicates incoherently, we do not recognize that there is a rich vein of experience comprising her past life. This other
dimension (that of life history) complements the social dimension to provide
a rounded personality.

Mental illness, however, adds another insidious barrier to communication
because older people with mental health problems suffer from what can be
described as multiple disadvantage. First, due to old age, comes the stereotyping of age-appropriate attitudes and behaviour. Secondly they suffer the
disadvantage of being mentally ill and the stigma that this still brings, as well
as the possibility that they will have some physical disability. Although this
appears to be a catalogue of disadvantages we are often unaware of their importance. Nurses, as members of society, will have the same attitudes and
prejudices as the rest of the population, but these are not always apparent
due to their subtle nature and their possible denial. Consequently, an understanding of the perceptions and social construction of old age and the implications for the individual are crucial to providing high quality nursing care.

It has been common in the past to treat the health condition, to view
patients as a collection of symptoms to be treated, rather than to view them as
rounded personalities. Fortunately, in mental health services, there is now
more credence given to a person-centred approach, but often this does not
go far enough. To gain a better insight into the needs of patients, it is necessary to understand their life history, the issues and events that moulded their
lives, which, in turn, reflect the social, economic and political circumstances
or environment in which they have lived.

To begin this process we need to examine the make-up of the elderly
population today and recognize any trends that this demonstrates, and the
implications that it has.

The demography of old age

The ageing population in the UK today is very different from that of the past,
brought about by the great social upheaval at the turn of the century. It is

important for us to recognize these changes, not only because many older people alive today will have experienced most of them first hand, but also because they are the basis for some assumptions about care and therefore may also affect the way in which we view older people.

When studying the demography of older people it is important to define what is meant by the words 'old' or 'older'. Statistical data can vary depending on how they are categorized. For example, some studies count everyone aged over sixty years, others over sixty-five. Some differentiate between younger and older age bands, but even here the parameters may be different. Although exact figures are important we are concerned here with trends and specific facets relating to sociological groups, such as sex, health or social conditions.

At the beginning of the twentieth century there were around two million people of what we would now describe as pensionable age. The data from the 1991 Census suggest that this has now increased to around 11.6 million, almost six times that in 1900. There has also been a marked increase in the proportion of the population who are older, from five per cent at the turn of the century to twenty-one per cent today (Office of Population Censuses and Surveys, 1993). The reason for this relates to two main factors: a decline in fertility and a decline in mortality.

In simple terms, since 1974 there have been less people born in the UK than are needed to replace the existing population. Choice is now much more influential in fertility; birth control, social influences and life style all affect the decision whether or not to have children, and the choice nowadays is usually for less children or none at all.

Declining mortality relates to both biological causes, such as medical developments, and sociological causes, such as increased standards of living and health care. These are very general observations, for, as we shall see later, quality of life is not the same for everyone. Another key sociological factor relating to mortality is the changing balance between the sexes, with about two out of three older people alive today being women. Marital status also illustrates a difference of gender, for, although over three-quarters of men aged sixty-five to seventy-four years are married, only half of the women in this age group are in a similar position. Consequently, it can be seen that most married women will be widowed for a greater part of their later life.

Generally speaking, the incidence of poverty rises with age. Among those aged over sixty-five years, around twenty-five per cent will be below Income Support level. Poverty is higher in older women than in men and is most common among those who have had manual jobs. Retirement nearly always results in a loss of income and the major part of a person's income is then likely to come from state benefits. Research shows that those who were involved in professional or managerial occupations receive almost half of their retirement income from occupational pensions and savings, compared with about five per cent in manual jobs (Victor and Evandrou, 1987). These factors seem to indicate that the differences in earlier life (class and occupation) have a direct influence on conditions in retirement, which in turn reflects on health status, including that of mental health. Similarly, there is an increasing trend for people to live alone; presently, this is more likely to be in rented than in owner-occupied accommodation. In many cases, housing conditions are likely to be worse for older people (Office of Population Censuses and Surveys, 1993).

It is not difficult to relate these effects to economic factors. The lack of occupational pension schemes for manual workers and the lack of recognition of women in the workforce are examples. It will be interesting to observe how these trends are affected in the future by such factors as major changes in retirement pension provision and a 'retired' workforce who may never have had a permanent job.

Ill health in old age is less common than is assumed, but the fear of being ill is a major concern in later life (Bearon, 1989). Good health has also been found to be the most important factor in predicting life satisfaction (Palmore and Kivett, 1977). Numerical information relating to mental health is also difficult to predict accurately, as this is often affected by what definition is given to particular conditions; for example commonly quoted data put the incidence of dementia for those aged over 65 as being ten per cent, rising to twenty per cent. Studies have also highlighted the increased incidence of mental health problems among women. Milne (1985) found, for example, that women were twice as likely to suffer from depressive illnesses than men, and that women were more likely to suffer from dementia.

Theories of ageing

The study of demography is not just an objective review of statistical changes, the interpretation of such data, as we have seen in the brief summary above, suggests cause and effect in the way that society, and older people within it, have developed. These theories put older people in a particular context which has changed over the years, reflecting different perspectives of interpretation. Two theories in particular have influenced popular economic and political thinking in this area. They are demographic transition theory and modernization theory.

Demographic transition theory

This 'traditional' theory suggests that the significant population changes that have occurred during this century are the result of a move from a rural to an industrial society. The consequence of this is that, whereas, in the past older people were respected and revered within an extended family, they have now become marginalized by a change in culture to which it has been difficult to adapt (Parsons 1942; Burgess, 1960). Not suprisingly, this model has been criticized for its oversimplification of the very complex changes in society that have occurred over the years.

Modernization theory

Similarly, modernization theory focuses on the move from rural agriculture to urban industrialization. Its main hypothesis is that the status of older people declines as the degree of modernization in a society increases (Cowgill and Holmes, 1972). In this process, the four areas of lowered status – health technology, economic technology, urbanization and education – are particularly significant. As with the theory of demographic transition, it tends to oversimplify. The key concept is a move from 'good' to 'bad', but to accept this we need to examine a few basic assumptions about old age in history.

The social theory of old age

Work since the 1950s has followed two major standpoints: the functionalist perspective and the political economy perspective.

Functionalist perspective

Just after World War II, the prevalent view in research was that old age was a social problem. The essence of these arguments related to the rapid changes that society was experiencing, where younger people were in an economically stronger position than they had been before. The 1960s with its new-found focus on youth also brought about a decline in the acceptance of the positive contribution of older people to society. Examples of factors that had produced problems for older people were the introduction of compulsory retirement; and increased mobility, which led to the rise of the nuclear family, where grown-up children left the area for work, creating their own insular family unit, gradually reducing the size of the family at home. The growth of industrialization and new technology, it is suggested, created a world with which older people could not identify.

This also fostered the myth of a golden age, which was superseded by a new order in which older people could no longer cope. The importance of this theory is that older people were seen as the problem, because they did not relate to the new environment. It should not be assumed, however, that older people were always viewed in a negative light. Some of the political thinking of the 1960s and 1970s recognized that society had a responsibility to its older members. The overriding view, however, was the paternalistic perception of a passive victim.

These theories relied very much on the assumption that people had roles in society. For example, if a man whose role had been to work for fifty years of his life, adjustment to retirement would mean a change of role, or, to be more precise a roleless role, a situation in which many individuals would find it difficult to cope. It is not surprising then that a large amount of research based on this model centres around peoples' inability to spend their time productively in retirement.

The other main functionalist model that appeared in the early 1960s is disengagement theory. This is usually attributed to Cumming and Henry (1961), who based their model on a survey carried out on a sample of healthy people aged over fifty years, in Kansas, Missouri, USA. The sample was studied over a period of time and changes in behaviour were noted. Disengagement theory is based on the principle that, as people grow older, they withdraw from contact with others in their social system. This process is gradual, and is accompanied by an increased preoccupation with themselves until eventually: 'the equilibrium which existed in middle life between the individual and his society has given way to a new equilibrium characterised by a greater distance and an altered type of relationship' (Cumming and Henry, 1961, p. 14).

The assumption is that it is seen as a natural progression to become less interested in life – a kind of preparation for death – which means that when death occurs, the individual is less likely to be involved in tasks that are considered to be of value to society. This theory was criticized because other researchers felt that their experience did not bear out the concept of disengagement. In fact, it was felt that people were clearly unhappy with their loss of role. The work of Townsend (1973), Shanas and Sussman (1977) and Blau (1973) is typical of such views.

In reality, the evidence is not clear cut. In some people, disengagement does take place, in others it does not. One positive aspect of disengagement theory, however, is the recognition that society and its institutions can accelerate the phenomenon, thereby accepting that older people lack the power to influence events.

Political economy perspective

By comparison, political economy theory suggests that the labelling of older people as victims is misleading, and gives society an excuse not to address the issues of their powerlessness. It suggests that being old is not, or should not be, a problem, but that it is the current context in which older people live that causes the problem.

> A political economy perspective analyses inequalities of all kinds of re-sources – health, income, assets, access to informal and formal care – not in terms of individual variation, but as resulting from the power relations that structure society (Arber and Ginn, 1991, p. 1).

Those who support this model suggest that we should be working towards a political and economic solution that aims to prevent inequality, thereby allowing the positive aspects of old age to flourish. The model looks at similarities rather than differences in age groups.

Another common element, in the more interactive studies, is the use of cohorts. A cohort, in this context, is a number of people who are all born around the same period of time, in similar situations. For example, people born at the turn of the century would experience World War I in their late teens and early twenties, and, because many of the men were killed, many women never married. These women would now be in their nineties, and there would therefore be a large number of women reaching old age compared with men. The other important point about a cohort is that it identifies what could generally be described as a social culture. For example, before the introduction of the National Health Service, visits by the family doctor incurred a charge. As a result, the doctor was only called out as a last resort. Today, people of that cohort are still wary of calling the doctor, and tend to be less assertive about health care.

Old age as a women's issue?

It is difficult to study old age without recognizing that it has particular implications for women. As we have seen earlier when considering demography, there are more older women than older men, and this difference appears to be widening. For those aged over sixty-five, the last 80 years has shown an increase in their life expectancy. Whereas men can now on average expect to live until they are seventy-eight, women can expect to live until they are eighty-three (Cental Statistical Office, 1989). It is also clear that there has been an increase in solo living (Wall, 1984) during the same period, and, as the majority of those living on their own are likely to be women, it is likely to be women who will rely on the formal network of care services. This is as true of mental health services as of any other. These patients are more likely to be women than men.

Mental health in old age

Although we are concerned in this text with a person-centred approach, it is worth providing an overview of the common mental illnesses affecting older people. We are particularly concerned with those disorders that have social, rather than organic, causes, but it would be too simplistic to divide them strictly in this way because organic illnesses also have a sociological impact. *The International Classification of Diseases* (World Health Organization, 1992), recognizes the following types of mental illness experienced by older people:

Organic mental disorders (dementia)

Dementia affects around ten per cent of those aged over sixty-five. It is believed that organic mental disorders are caused by structural changes in the brain. The most common is Alzheimer's disease, but a large minority relate to the vascular dementias (vascular dementia of acute onset, multi-infarct dementia and subcortical vascular dementia). There are also a number of less common types of dementia.

Schizophrenia

Only a small number of older people (around one per cent) are affected by schizophrenia. When it manifests itself in old age it is generally as a paranoid illness, but it must also be remembered that younger people with schizophrenia will grow old and will require the support to meet the additional problems of old age.

Affective disorders

Manic symptoms generally appear in old age after a long period of recurrent depression, although other persistent mood disorders are also common.

Neurotic, stress related disorders

Just under ten per cent of people aged over sixty-five are thought to suffer from such disorders, although they are often unlikely to be recognized by GPs. The most common phobia in old age is agoraphobia, which can be particularly disabling because it leads to isolation of the individual.

Personality disorder

This is essentially long-term 'maladaptive behaviour'. It occurs in a variety of situations and is not necessarily old age-related. It should also be recognized that such behaviours can occur as a result of dementia.

Alcohol and drug-related disorders

There is a common misconception that alcohol abuse in not an issue for older people. Obviously there will be instances of chronic alcoholics who have survived to old age, but there is another group, particularly women, who develop alcohol problems in later life. Drug dependence is more difficult to define, as overreliance has to be balanced against the quality of life that pre-scribed drugs facilitate.

The social context of cause and effect

In following a medical model of nursing, cause and effect would generally seem to be physiological in nature, but mental health is heavily influenced by social factors, and the added dimension of old age creates specific areas of concern when attempting to identify appropriate nursing interventions.

Murphy (1982) found that major traumatic events in life are direct causes of depressive illnesses in old age. Similarly, social difficulties and poor health can add to this vulnerability, as can the lack of a supportive partner, family or friend. One of the most common, and most serious, causes of trauma in old age is bereavement.

Bereavement

Colin Murray Parkes, one of the foremost authorities on bereavement, de-scribed the bereavement process as passing through four stages (Parkes, 1986). These are: numbness, restlessness/pining, anger and resolution. It is at the third stage, when social withdrawal and mild depression are quite normal, that the situation may develop into severe depression with the risk of suicide. Wattis and Martin (1994) add another interesting observation:

> In men especially, the death rate from physical illness in the year following bereavement increases beyond chance expectation and three-quarters of these deaths are due to heart problems. People really do seem to die of a 'broken heart' (Wattis and Martin, 1994, pp. 75–76).

Health

Although evidence suggests that mortality amongst older people has decreased over the past twenty years (Office of Population Censuses and Surveys, 1990a), it is less clear whether this means there has been an increase in people experiencing healthier living within this period. The 'compression of morbidity theory' (Fries, 1980), for example, suggests that ill health is squeezed into the late years of life, thereby providing longer periods of activity and wellbeing. This may be true as a generalization, but we also know that individuals are affected by a number of other factors.

Arber and Ginn (1991) put forward a strong argument that gender and social class affect general health and that women and working class people are more prone to ill health. The general household survey offers ample statistical evidence relating to gender and ill health (Office of Population Censuses and Surveys, 1990b) and the work of Fox et al. (1983) and Goldblatt (1990) makes a correlation between health and social class. To test this hypothesis, think of your own patients/residents/clients with mental health problems. What is their gender, and from what social class do they come?

Psychological factors

One of the theories relating to the cause of depression in old age has developed from the concept of 'learned helplessness' formulated by Seligman (1975), who found that, if individuals are constantly traumatized by events over which they have no control, they eventually give up. This is clearly illustrated in the following extract:

> Compulsory retirement is usual in the UK, however good people are at their work and however much they may wish to continue... Physical disabilities may accumulate despite efforts to keep fit... Old friends may seem to die off at an alarming rate, providing a link between the learned helplessness theory, bereavement and depression (Wattis and Martin, 1994, p. 77).

When considering the social and environmental causes of ill health we cannot omit the area of organic mental disorders. This is because of the particularly stressful role this puts on carers of those people with such illnesses as dementia, making the carers themselves susceptible to mental ill health. There have been many studies around this topic, the best known being that carried out by Gilhooly (1984), who recognized the unusual behaviour of those with dementia as being a clear case of stress (for example, night wanderings, bizarre and dangerous behaviour, or demands for attention).

Others have suggested that it is the dementing person's mental state that causes more stress than their physical infirmities (Wheatley, 1979; Gilleard, 1982). Some key observations that nurses, particularly those working in the community, need to recognize, is that the carers themselves are often old and are not as demanding of services. They are often unaware of what is available to them.

Most studies also show that most carers tend to be daughters. The reasons for this are varied, but a major factor is still the expectation that the female members of the family will provide care.

Conclusion

In this chapter we have considered the demography of old age and the social construction of older persons in society. We have also examined the theories of the impact of social policy and its effects on older people, and the changing attitudes illustrated by the different theories regarding old age. What we now need to ensure is that this knowledge can be put into practice. The following are practical suggestions for nurses.

Develop a clearer understanding of social theory

Nurse training needs to attach more importance to the social context of care for all the reasons described above. Until this happens, a self-motivated start to understanding social history will be useful. Many resources are available which describe the social and economic history and give an insight into the society in which many older people have lived (1900–1950s). Do not forget that we live in a multicultural society and that a cultural and religious understanding of a person's background is essential. For a broader economic and political perspective, consider the publications and observations on the community care legislation and its implications.

Recommended reading for theory related to health care is *Gender and Later*

Life by Sara Arber and Jay Ginn (Arber and Ginn, 1991), and *The Sociology of Old Age* (Fennell et al. 1988). Both books include references to further sources.

Examine the local demographic perspective

Population statistics are available for each locality, but try any secondary sources that are available. For example, the social services department in your local authority may have collected statistics and produced reports that will be of use to you. (For example, my local social services department completed a survey of carers in the community. One surprising finding was that there were more male carers than the national average. This obviously had implications for the community psychiatric nursing service.) Nurses must be able to apply this knowledge in a practical situation.

Examine the life course perspective

The understanding of a life course perspective, especially regarding the characteristics of a group of a similar age in a similar situation (cohort), can be used in many ways. For example, at the time of writing, I have just returned from a hospital service to celebrate Remembrance Sunday. All members of the congregation participated in a meaningful way, despite the fact that some of them could be described as having severe organic impairment. This reminiscence therapy does not have to be on a grand scale but can relate to smaller events that would be common in everyday life (former occupation, or household chores, for example). It would be hoped that this information would be obtained on assessment, but some simple detective work on how old the persons were and what kind of background they came from would also be helpful.

Treat the person, not the symptoms

Older people do not suddenly become old. They have a clearly documented life history, which, if you are willing to look for it, will provide you with a basis for some high-quality nursing care. The observation of social behaviour both in the past and in the present will help to undermine some of the popular myths about old age, and hopefully prevent their further perpetuation in the working environment. More importantly, it will encourage nurses not only to recognize older people as individuals but also help them to act as advocates.

In this way, appropriate future care provision may be organized for these members of society who so far have had little opportunity to contribute to their own treatment and care in service planning.

References

Arber, S. and Ginn, J. (1991). *Gender and Later Life*. London: Sage.

Bearon, L. B. (1989). No great expectations: the underpinnings of life satisfaction for older women. *The Gerontologist*, **29**(6), 772–84.

Blau, Z. (1973). *Old Age in a Changing Society*. New York: New Viewpoints.

Burgess, E. W. (ed.) (1960). *Ageing in Western Societies*. Chicago: University of Chicago Press.

Central Statistical Office (1989). *Social Trends 19*. London: HMSO.

Cowgill, D. O. and Holmes, D. (eds) (1972). *Ageing and Modernization*. New York: Appleton.

Cumming, E. and Henry, W. E. (1961). *Growing Old, the Process of Disengagement*. New York: Basic Books.

Fennell, G., Phillipson, C. and Evers, H. (1988). *The Sociology of Old Age*. Milton Keynes: Open University.

Fox, A. J., Goldblatt, P. and Jones, D. R. (1983). *Social Class Mortality Differentials from the OPCS Longitudinal Study 1971–75*. London: HMSO.

Fries, J. F. (1980). Ageing, natural death and the compression of morbidity. *New England Journal of Medicine*, **303**(3), 130–35.

Gilhooly, M. L. M. (1984). The impact of care giving on care-givers. *British Journal of Medical Psychology*, **37**, 35–44.

Gilleard, C. L. (1982). *Stresses and Strains amongst Supporters of the Elderly Infirm Day Hospital Attenders*. Edinburgh: University of Edinburgh.

Goldblatt, P. (1990). *Mortality and Social Organization in England and Wales, 1971–81*. London: HMSO.

Milne, J. (1985). *Clinical Effects of Ageing: a Longitudinal Study*. London: Croom Helm.

Murphy, E. (1982). The social origins of depression in old age. *British Journal of Psychiatry*, **141**, 135–142.

Office of Population Censuses and Surveys (1990a) *Population Trends*, 61. London: HMSO.

Office of Population Censuses and Surveys (1990). *Mortality Statistics, 1987. England and Wales DH1 No. 20*. London: HMSO.

Office of Population Censuses and Surveys (1993). *Census 1991, National Report, Great Britain*. London: HMSO.

Palmore, E. B. and Kivett, V. (1997). Change in life satisfactions: a longitudinal study of persons 46–70. *Journal of Gerontology*, **32**(3), 311–16.

Parkes, C. M. (1986). *Bereavement: Studies of Grief in Adult Life*. London: Pelican.

Parsons, T. (1942). Age and sex in the social structure of the United States. *American Sociological Review*, **7**, 604–16.

Seligman, M. E. (1975). *Helplessness: on Depression, Development and Death*. San Francisco; Freeman.

Shanas, E. and Sussman, M. B. (eds) (1977). *Family Bureaucracy and the Elderly*. Durham NC publishers, Duke University Press.

Townsend, P. (1973). *The Social Minority*. London: Allen Lane.

Victor, C. and Evandrou, M. (1987). Does Social Class Matter in Later Life? In *Social Gerontology: New Directions*. S. di Gregoria (ed.), pp. 252–267, London: Croom Helm.

Wall, R. (1948). Residential isolation of the elderly, a comparison over time. *Ageing and Society*, **4**, 483–503.

Wattis, J. and Martin, C. (1994). Practical Psychiatry of Old Age, 2nd ed. London: Chapman & Hall.

Wheatley, V. (1979). *Supporters of Elderly Persons with a Dementing Illness Living in the Same Household*. Guildford: University of Surrey.

World Health Organisation (1992). *The ICD10 Classification of Mental and Behavioural Disorders; Clinical Descriptions and Diagnostic Guidelines*. Geneva: WHO.

3

Mental illness in old age

Tracey Sharp

Introduction

This chapter provides an overview of the major mental health problems facing older people in the UK today. Although subsequent chapters explore these problems and the appropriate nursing interventions in greater detail, this chapter will set these in context with a general introduction to mental illness in old age, explaining some of the reasons why this occurs.

A quasi-medical approach is adopted, describing the clinical features of the mental illnesses commonly diagnosed in old age. Consideration is also given to the various methods of assessment used to detect the presence and extent of mental illness, and to the appropriate interventions that nurses may make.

The overall aim of the chapter is to equip readers with an understanding of the most prevalent mental health problems found in older people and the reasons why these occur.

Background

Old age is generally considered to begin between the ages of sixty and sixty-five years. At this time in their lives, society's expectations of older people begin to change, and generalizations are made about their seemingly diminishing capabilities. Stereotypes then develop of the 'elderly' person as a non-productive member of society, who will become increasingly ill, immobile and 'feeble-minded'. Indeed, many stereotypes seem to portray mental health problems, and in particular dementia, as being an inevitable consequence of ageing. However, it is important to make clear that not all older people suffer mental health problems and, of those who do, not everyone will suffer from dementia.

Adjustments to ageing

With ageing comes inevitable change. However, people's responses to such change and the ways in which they adapt are highly individualized. Although some are able to function well during times of change, others may cope less well.

Physical change

Ageing is likely to bring with it a decline in the senses, such as hearing, taste, smell and sight. There are also visible changes including a loss in height, wrinkling of the skin, and greying and thinning of the hair. Reduced motility of the digestive system may lead to constipation and poor absorption of nutrients, while the kidneys become less efficient in filtering waste and toxins from the blood. In addition, there may be cardiovascular and respiratory changes, accompanied by joint weakness and decreased mobility. The health survey for England (HMSO, 1991), reported that sixty-four per cent of men and fifty-nine per cent of women over the age of sixty-five suffer a long-standing illness or disability, usually of a musculoskeletal nature.

Social change

Retirement is likely to bring with it reduced income. This, when coupled with ill health and declining mobility, can make socializing more difficult. In addition, reduced productivity and the older person's perceived usefulness in society may be hard for many to come to terms with. Such role changes can lead to feelings of low self-esteem and self-worth.

Ageing is also a time of loss and bereavement. The death of friends or a spouse will inevitably result in an increasing awareness of one's own mortality, along with fewer opportunities for socialization. It is also likely that children will have grown up and left home with the further possibility of role reversal with older children having begun to care for the parent(s).

Psychological change

Ageing produces changes in the brain, with a reduction in the number of functioning neurones and in cerebral weight. However, despite much research, the effect of these changes upon mental functioning is unclear (Rabins, 1992) and individualized. Although some do suffer a decline in cognitive processes such as recall and recognition, and the speed with which they can perform tasks, for others there may be only minimal loss.

Mental illness in old age

According to the 1991 Census, the UK has an estimated nine million people over the age of sixty-five. While currently representing 15.7% of the population this is expected to rise to twenty-two per cent by the year 2031 (Office for National Statistics, 1994). Clearly, one inevitable consequence of this ageing population will be a greater demand for the provision of health care. Already, just over one-third of all admissions to mental illness beds are for those over the age of sixty-five (Department of Health, 1992a).

The presence of mental illness in old age is broadly classified as being either organic or functional. The term organic is used to describe those illnesses for which a physical cause and explanation can be established. However, this distinction is becoming blurred due to recent discoveries of biochemical abnormalities in those suffering from so-called 'functional' illnesses such as depression (Murphy, 1992) and schizophrenia.

Outlined below are the most common diagnoses made for these two types of mental illness, with descriptions of presenting signs and symptoms.

Organic illness

Organic illness can be further divided into those that are reversible (or acute states) and those that are irreversible and progressive. Reversible states if detected and treated quickly, can result in a return to normal life style. However, progressive states, such as the dementias, lead ultimately to an early death.

Acute confusional states

Acute confusional states may also be referred to as delirium. The confusion appears rapidly, perhaps over a period of hours, with a sudden deterioration in the person's mental state. The main features are clouding of consciousness and disorientation, which may be accompanied by hallucinations, anxiety, restlessness and agitation. The symptoms are likely to be worse at night. Although confusion is considered in greater detail in other chapters, some of its more common causes are described below.

Ageing can affect the ways in which medications are absorbed by the body, due to fluctuations in the excretion and metabolism of drugs. The increasing volume and range of medication prescribed for physical illnesses can, therefore, without careful monitoring, produce confusional states. Certain types of medication or their sudden withdrawal can also cause confusion.

Confusion may arise from sources of *infection*, especially of the respiratory and urinary tracts. This is usually accompanied by pyrexia.

Metabolic and endocrine disorders may cause acute confusion. These include disorders such as hypothyroidism, diabetes and renal failure. Confusion can also result from electrolyte and fluid imbalance due to dehydration or malnutrition, and from vitamin B deficiencies (Bayer, 1991).

Confusion can result from *trauma*, including damage to the brain from head injuries or cerebrovascular accidents. Such trauma may be reversible or cause permanent damage.

Physical illness or disease that interrupts the blood or oxygen supply to the brain can produce *anoxia* resulting in confusion, for example, respiratory or cardiac failure.

Neoplasm can cause the destruction of brain cells while obstructing the flow of blood and cerebrospinal fluid. Symptoms differ according to the location but there is often a change in personality, clouding of consciousness or memory failure. Further signs of neoplasm include headaches, dizziness, vomiting, bradycardia and papilloedema.

The diagnosis of *alcoholism* in older people can be difficult because problems can be masked by the changes of ageing. Cognitive impairment from alcohol can be difficult to distinguish from other confusional states, while the poor management of personal affairs may simply be attributed to forgetfulness or fatigue (Gambert and Hartford, 1991).

There is a steep rise in the incidence of newly diagnosed cases of *epilepsy* over the age of fifty years. The commonest causes of this are cerebrovascular disease and the presence of cerebral tumours (Tallis, 1992).

Finally, confusion may also arise from *unfamiliar surroundings*; older people who are admitted to hospital can quickly become disorientated. Postoperative confusion may also be experienced by those who have undergone surgery. Indeed, it has been estimated that one in four elderly patients admitted to a general hospital will suffer some degree of confusion at some point in their stay (Lipowski, 1992).

Dementias

Dementia is thought to affect five per cent of people over the age of 65 and twenty per cent of those over the age of eighty years (Department of Health, 1992b). Following the onset, life expectancy is between four and twelve years.

The Working Party on Care of the Dementing Elderly (1988) has defined dementia as: 'an acquired global impairment of intellect, memory, and personality without the impairment of consciousness. It is almost always of long duration, usually progressive and irreversible.'

Dementia can result from many factors, including some of those outlined in the previous section (e.g. trauma and infection); however, the key symptoms of all dementias, to a greater or lesser degree, are contained in four main areas (Norman, 1991a).

There will be *cognitive* changes. Short-term memory impairment is evident with thought and speech content that is dominated by the past. Confabulation may be present, which is used by the person to fill in memory gaps. Judgement and understanding become impaired with a general inability to grasp situations fully and to respond accordingly. Disorientation in time, place and person occurs, together with restlessness, which may be worse at night.

There may be a lack of *emotional* control with catastrophic reactions of anger, hostility or despair when pushed beyond the limits of their ability. Mood changes may be evident with symptoms of anxiety and depression. This may be accompanied by paranoia and suspicion of any change. When combined with forgetfulness, this can typically lead sufferers to accuse others of theft.

Social problems will become evident. Competence in self-care declines and difficulties are experienced in normal activities of living such as cooking, shopping and cleaning. This deteriorates later into a complete disregard for personal hygiene and self-care. Restlessness and wandering can occur in addition to uninhibited and antisocial behaviour such as incontinence, public undressing and aggression. Communication and speech become increasingly difficult as well as the ability to follow conversations.

The *physical* appearance can change, with seemingly rapid ageing. General physical deterioration occurs as the dementia develops, with the person becoming gradually more helpless. Finally, he or she may fall prey to physical illness and infection. Pneumonia is a frequent cause of death.

Alzheimer's disease
This is the most common and probably the most well known of the dementias. It embraces the majority of the symptoms described above. The Alzheimer's Disease Society (1993), estimate that, within the UK there are almost 636 000 people with dementia and of these, nearly half a million will have Alzheimer's disease. A definite diagnosis can only be made during post-mortem examination.

Despite the vast amount of research into Alzheimer's disease in recent years, its cause remains unclear. Studies have considered genetic factors, abnormal protein structures, toxins such as aluminium, infections, and the absence of certain neurotransmitters within the brain (Burnside, 1988; Nelson, 1990). However, these findings have been inconclusive and unable to explain every instance of Alzheimer's disease. More recently it has been suggested that it is the cumulative effect of these factors that results in neuronal loss (Tobiansky, 1993).

Arteriosclerotic dementia or multi-infarct dementia

This vascular dementia is the second most common cause of dementia, and is responsible for up to twenty per cent of cases (Friedland, 1992). It is caused by impaired circulation to the brain resulting in cerebral infarcts. Each infarct produces a period of memory loss and impaired consciousness. Key features are its abrupt onset, with a sudden decline in cognitive ability as well as behavioural changes. This is followed by a plateau lasting for a period of days or weeks (Tobiansky, 1994a). Further neurological signs may be present such as paralysis, aphasia, apraxia and convulsions.

Parkinson's disease

There is significant overlap in the pathology of Parkinson's disease with that of Alzheimer's disease and studies have found the incidence of dementia in up to twenty per cent of patients suffering from Parkinson's disease (Hildick-Smith, 1991). However, this is primarily a motor disorder with patients displaying a stooped posture, a fine tremor, a shuffling gait, muscle weakness and rigidity.

Lewy body disease

Until recently, this was considered to be very rare. It is thought to be a variant of Alzheimer's disease, but it also has parkinsonian features such as rigidity, tremor and a shuffling gait. Hallucinations and delusions are more evident than in Alzheimer's disease (Tobiansky, 1994b).

HIV-related dementia

This condition is likely to be caused by direct infection of the central nervous system by HIV. Its incidence is expected to rise in older people, given the increasing numbers aged over sixty years with HIV and AIDS (Marr, 1994). The AIDS dementia complex closely resembles Alzheimer's disease, although its progress is more rapid. Symptoms include depression, agitation, delusions, hallucinations and paranoia. Neurological features are also likely be present, such as numbness in the limbs, headaches and seizures (Ebersole and Hess, 1990).

Creutzfeldt–Jakob disease
This has become more well known due to media attention, which has focused on its relationship with scrapie, a disease of sheep and goats (Livingston, 1994). It is thought to be transmitted by a virus and is rapidly progressive, with death expected within one year of onset. Other neurological symptoms occur such as illusions, hallucinations, muscle wasting and blindness (Nelson, 1990).

Pick's disease
This disease is rare, accounting for only one to two per cent of all those diagnosed with dementia (Bayer, 1991). Although Pick's disease is similar to Alzheimer's disease, brain cell loss is focused in the frontal and temporal lobes. Consequently, behavioural changes are more evident, with diminished control over impulses and inhibitions. There may also be mood changes and lack of emotional stability. However, although there is a progressive decline in the sufferer's personality there may be little intellectual or memory loss.

Functional illness

Functional illnesses include the affective disorders such as depression and mania, schizophrenia-type psychoses, neuroses and personality disorders.

Depression

Depression is described as a unipolar affective disorder. Although its prevalence would appear to be no higher than in younger adults (Henderson, 1992), it is thought to be the most common functional illness found in old age (Brayne and Ames, 1988). For those who first experience it in old age, it is likely to occur within the setting of a physical illness (Jolley and Jolley, 1991). Indeed, one survey of physically ill older people found that twenty per cent were suffering clinically significant depression (O'Riordan et al., 1989).

Depression can present with affective, biological and cognitive symptoms (Burn and Drearden, 1990).

- Affective
  Prominent and persistent low mood
  Loss of interest and pleasure (in self and surroundings)
  Diurnal variation of mood

- Biological
    Loss of appetite and weight
    Sleep disturbance with early morning wakening
    Reduced energy
    Psychomotor agitation or retardation
- Cognitive
    Ideas of worthlessness and guilt
    Reduced concentration
    Thoughts of death or suicide
    Hallucinations and delusions

In older people, diagnosis is made difficult due to the ways in which the presenting symptoms can be misinterpreted. For example, the depression may be complicated by the presence of somatic complaints, obsessional behaviour or hypochondria. In addition, although depression is frequently associated with psychomotor retardation, in older people there may be increased activity and agitation with aimless wandering both day and night.

When the depression is profound, there may be cognitive impairment and confusion which can be misdiagnosed as dementia. Nihilistic delusions may also be present with complete self-neglect resulting in malnutrition, dehydration, muteness and withdrawal or stupor.

Depression also carries with it an increased risk of suicide. Men over the age of seventy-five consistently have the highest suicide rate in the UK compared with other age groups (Department of Health, 1992b). Risk factors associated with suicidal behaviour include the presence of depression, physical illness, social isolation, alcohol abuse and recent contact with primary care services (Lindesay, 1993).

Mania and manic-depressive illness

The presence of manic-depressive illness (a bipolar affective disorder) is unlikely to occur for the first time in old age. More usually, it is a recurrence of symptoms from early life. Sufferers appear overly cheerful, overactive and noisy, sometimes spilling over into aggressive behaviour. If the condition is untreated, the person can become exhausted through lack of sleep and may suffer dehydration and malnutrition.

Schizophrenia and paraphrenia

Schizophrenia that is suffered throughout life tends to become less intense with age and it is comparatively rare for it to develop for the first time in old age (Riley, 1990). However, paraphrenia may occur. This is a form of late-onset schizophrenia manifesting with marked paranoid symptoms and persecutory delusions. It is most common among elderly women who live alone, and who may believe that they are being spied upon or that neighbours are plotting or conspiring against them. Hallucinations may also be present.

Other mental health problems

Other mental illnesses, such as the neuroses and personality disorders are not fully discussed here, although chronic neurotic disorders that have developed early in life are thought to lessen with age (Bergman, 1992). Symptoms of hypochondria and obsessional behaviour which are more common in old age (Riley, 1990), should be fully investigated for evidence of organic illness or for underlying depressive symptoms.

Assessment

The mental health of older people can be affected by many factors, each interwoven to form a complex relationship. Acute confusional states are often compounded by social elements that need to be fully assessed along with the underlying physical illness. For example, pain and reduced mobility may discourage an older person from cooking and preparing food. In addition, there may be limited social or family support to ensure checks upon the person's wellbeing and ability to meet his or her nutritional needs. Ultimately, such poor eating habits could lead to malnourishment, dehydration and subsequent confusion.

A failure to assess such factors fully may result in erroneous diagnoses based purely upon the presenting signs and symptoms, while the contributory physical and social elements remain unaddressed. Most confusional states are reversible if treated promptly and appropriately, although, if they are overlooked, they can become progressive and irreversible. Assessment should therefore be of the whole person and not just of the illness and the presenting problems.

First contact

The GP contract introduced in April 1990 committed family practitioners to screen annually all those patients on their list who are over the age of seventy-five years. Screening includes a review of the home environment and discussion with relatives and carers when appropriate. In addition, social, mobility, continence, mental, functional, hearing and vision assessments are made, along with a review of any medication. Such screening is frequently delegated to community nurses, although questions have been raised regarding the effectiveness and appropriateness of this (Garrett, 1992). Its value may also be limited when elderly people consider this to be an invasion of their privacy and are reluctant to report their health care needs.

More frequently, the person's needs will come to light following an approach to the GP by a concerned carer or neighbour, or from calls to the police or the emergency services once problems have reached serious proportions. A typical scenario is of a confused elderly person who is found wandering the streets at night, or, after having fallen and sustained an injury, is requiring attendance at an accident and emergency department. Referrals are then made to a psychiatrist or community psychiatric nurse.

Planning the assessment

Assessment may be undertaken either in the older person's home, following inpatient admission, or at a day hospital. Although the location may be dependent upon the severity of the illness, the assessment of the person within the home environment will be necessary at some point in order to determine his or her level of functioning there, and to gauge the individual's life style, daily routine and levels of support. In addition, it must be recognized that the unfamiliar surroundings of a hospital can exacerbate disorientation and give a false impression of a person's abilities. Therefore, assessments carried out in a health care setting should aim to be as comfortable and homely as possible, while being quiet and free from distraction.

Assessment is likely to involve a range of professionals, each assessing particular aspects of the patient's needs. For example: the occupational therapist and the physiotherapist may assess the patient's independence and functioning at home; the social worker may determine the patient's and the carer's financial entitlements; the psychologist may assess cognitive ability through formal psychological testing; the nurse may assess the need for emotional support, education and development of coping strategies for both the patient and the carer, while the doctor may prescribe medication for the alleviation of symptoms.

Multidisciplinary teams work together in a number of ways. Some may examine referrals within team conferences, allocating a keyworker who can best respond to that person's needs. Others may prefer referrals to be made to a psychiatrist, who will diagnose and begin medical treatment before deciding upon the appropriate involvement of other team members.

Assessment may include open-ended questioning during informal interviews, structured question and answer tests, rating scales or observation of behaviour. Above all, it is important to develop a warm, nonthreatening rapport with the person. Good communication skills are essential to reduce anxiety and encourage willingness to participate in the assessment (Farran and Keane-Haggerty, 1989).

Undertaking the assessment

There are many diverse assessment tools that can be used to measure all aspects of physical, mental and social functioning. Many are reviewed by Burnside (1988), Ebersole and Hess (1990), Hogstel (1990), Kane and Bayer (1991), Norman (1991b) and Yurick et al. (1989); however, there is no single measure that is universally appropriate to every patient.

Although some assessment may be made early during history-taking, further assessments may only be possible over time with repeated visits or following admission to hospital, when continuous observation may be made by nursing staff.

History
History-taking should gather information relating to the presenting complaint and the sequence of events prior to this. It should include the incidence of past psychiatric illness, both in the person concerned and the family, and whether there have been any recent physical illnesses, injuries or major life events. Each of these can help to determine the speed of onset of the symptoms and identify likely indicators for the presenting illness.

Assessment should aim to determine what is normal for the person, so that deviations from the norm can be detected. Exploration should be made of the patient's usual routines of daily living and coping skills, and how these have been affected by the illness.

Some people may find it difficult to communicate, or may confabulate and provide inaccurate information. In these cases, it will be necessary to obtain further details and confirmation of the history from a range of sources. This may include carers, relatives, friends and neighbours, or other health professionals. If the person is in hospital, then details may be gleaned from escorts at the time of admission or from visiting relatives; otherwise it may be necessary to enlist the help of the social work department or a community psychiatric nurse.

Physical problems

As mental health problems in old age are frequently associated with physical illness, it is necessary to undertake a full physical examination with a review of medication as well as an electrocardiogram, and electroencephalogram, skull and chest radiographs, and blood and urine tests. Such assessments help to exclude any physical causes of confusion arising from infection, neoplasm or polypharmacy. For example, although pyrexia may indicate infection, hypertension may signify the presence of multi-infarct dementia. The assessment of hearing and sight can help to explain reasons for paranoia.

It is also important to determine what is the person's main concern and what impact any physical ill health may have upon their life style. Are there problems with breathing, eating, elimination or sleeping? Has there been a loss of appetite and weight? Does physical disability mean that the person is unable to care for him or herself?

Psychological and mental assessment

The assessment of cognitive ability and mood can be made by both listening to and observing the person. Speech rate and content can provide clues to mental wellbeing. For example, does the person speak in monosyllables or does he or she ramble and appear confused? Does the content indicate anxiety, fear, paranoia or feelings of worthlessness? Is the person irritable, hostile or aggressive? Does the individual appear to be deluded or to be responding to hallucinations?

Observation of the person's behaviour, body language and facial expression also gives clues to the mental state. Is the person wandering about and pacing the floor? Does the individual look depressed or happy? Is there an inability to concentrate on tasks and follow a conversation? Is there any disorientation to time, place and person?

Formal screening tests may be used to determine both mood and cognitive impairment. However, these need to be administered by someone who is familiar with the test used and is able to interpret the results. Screening tests may include the assessment of memory (recent and remote), concentration, mood, suicidal risk, judgement, problem solving, intelligence, reasoning, general knowledge and orientation.

Social and functional assessment

These assessments should ideally take place in the home environment and should examine the person's independence in all activities of daily living, such as personal hygiene, safety, mobility and nutrition. Many indicators can be gained from observing the condition of a person's house and garden, and also the individual's general appearance and behaviour, such as the state of his or her dress, hair and teeth, and evidence of continence. The assessment of functional ability can identify the need for various levels of support and for aids and adaptations to the home environment.

It is also necessary to examine the person's social network, any recreational activities and support from friends and carers as well as other agencies (i.e. social services). If the person is living alone, is he or she able to shop, wash, housekeep and manage money? What are the living conditions like? Is there adequate heating? Are there safety hazards? In assessing these skills and conditions, however, one needs to be aware of gender divisions and the fact that some men may never have learned to perform certain tasks.

Dementia versus depression

The value of good assessment is evident in being able to determine the difference between dementia and depression. As noted earlier, these illnesses can present with similar features, although they require different nursing and medical interventions. It is important not to confuse the symptoms of depression with dementia and to be aware that patients in the early stages of dementia often have depressive symptoms (Burns et al., 1990), while those who are depressed frequently complain of memory failure (Murphy, 1992). Misdiagnosis is common. For example, the apathy experienced in depression may result in the person responding to questions with 'don't know' answers which may be interpreted as a sign of forgetfulness or of cognitive impairment.

Assessment should therefore examine both the affective and cognitive symptoms experienced by the person. In dementia, assessment and intervention can delay dependency, while for depression, early detection and treatment can alleviate symptoms while reducing the risk of suicide.

With depression, the onset is more likely to have been recent: a matter of months rather than years. History-taking may also uncover experiences of depression in early life or a family history of depressive illness. Typical presenting symptoms may include a depressed mood, expressed feelings of hopelessness, and disturbed eating and sleeping patterns (Robins, 1984). In contrast, confused people are more likely to have some element of over-activity than those who are depressed.

Treatment and interventions

Assessment does, of course, lead to care planning using interventions appropriate to the problems that have been identified. Although specific interventions are explored in greater detail in subsequent chapters, ultimately, the nurse's role is to help the older person and the carers to adapt and to live in their preferred environment for as long as possible. The nurse can facilitate this by employing various caring and coping strategies that can alleviate the stress and anxiety experienced by both sufferers and carers.

Admission to hospital

Initially, admission to hospital may be necessary to enable close observation and a full assessment of the person's condition and problems. The decision to do this may also be made to provide respite for carers. However, if possible, it is best to treat older people in their own home so that hospital admission does not exacerbate further confusion or paranoia. Support in the community may be provided by community psychiatric nurses, GPs, home helps, meals on wheels, and other voluntary organizations.

Day hospitals may be used to combine the need for a continuing assessment of the person and giving daily respite to carers, while allowing access to the care provided by other health professionals such as chiropodists and physiotherapists. At this time, treatment and management routines adopted by staff can be continued by carers in the home environment.

Medication

Appropriate medication may be prescribed for those suffering from confusional states arising from infection. For others who have disturbed sleep or restless behaviour, mild hypnotics or sedatives can be given, while depression may be alleviated by antidepressants supported by a range of psychological interventions. The use of medication needs to be considered carefully, to reduce the risk of drug interactions or difficulties in the person's metabolism, which may exacerbate the presenting problem (Knopman and Sawyer-DeMaris, 1990). There may also be difficulties in ensuring compliance with treatment, particularly in those who are confused or when there are complicated drug schedules. Bottles should be clearly labelled with clear instructions, although the nurse may also need to explain the times and dosages and write these down if appropriate.

Psychological approaches

Psychological approaches may be used with those who are confused, including reality orientation, validation and reminiscence. For those who are suffering functional illnesses, anxiety management and related cognitive therapies may be considered (Conway, 1988). Such interventions may be held either on a one-to-one basis or in groups, with support and interaction encouraged from other group members.

Both at home and in other settings, daily activities that are repetitive may help to reduce disorientation and anxiety from failing memory. The establishment of routines gives structure to each day.

Encouragement should also be given to the person to remain independent for as long as possible, while adequate time is given to them to perform their activities. At all times, emphasis should be placed upon the person's abilities rather than on their disabilities. Following functional assessment, aids to assist in the maintenance of self-care and promote safety may include walking frames, bath seats, toilet seat raisers, chair raise blocks, shoe horns, special cutlery and kitchen equipment.

Support for carers

Support is also needed by carers, who are frequently old themselves. Caring can be exhausting and demoralizing, and can cause grief and depression in the carers themselves. Often, they are distressed because they do not understand the patient's illness and behaviour, or they feel unsupported and helpless. An exploration of their needs is important and counselling may also be required, together with advice on coping and the management strategies that can be adopted. Further support can also be given by carers groups.

Overall, the nurse needs to assume an educational and a supportive role, towards both the older person and any significant others. In order to do this effectively, it is important to develop a good rapport and trusting relationship that demonstrates the nurse's real interest and concern in the wellbeing of both the person and their carers.

Conclusion

This chapter has provided an introduction to the range of mental health problems that may face older people. It has set these in the context of the inevitable changes and adjustments that an older person must make to ageing and the physical ageing process. Two broad classifications of mental illness have been identified: organic and functional. Organic illnesses are those for which a physical cause is evident; they may be reversible (acute confusion rising from infection) or progressive (dementias). The main functional illness affecting older people is depression, carrying with it a high risk of suicide. Careful assessment is needed to determine the cause of mental illness in older people due to the complex interplay between physical illnesses, social factors and the confusing presenting signs and symptoms; misdiagnosis is common. The assessment of an older person should involve all members of the multidisciplinary team and should gather information from a range of sources. Communication skills are vital to ensuring the participation of the sufferers and their carers in the assessment and planning of care. Treatment and interventions for specific problems are explored in subsequent chapters, through the use of medication, psychological and cognitive therapies, education and the provision of aids to daily living.

References

Alzheimer's Disease Society. (1993). *Deprivation in Dementia*. London: ADS.

Bayer, A. J. (1991). Cognitive impairment – diagnosis and management. In *Principles and Practice of Geriatric Medicine*. (M. S. J. Pathy, ed.) pp. 933–951. Chichester: Wiley.

Bergman, K. (1992). Functional psychiatric disorders in old age. In *Oxford Textbook of Geriatric Medicine*. (J. G. Evans and T. F. Williams, eds.) pp. 634–638. Oxford: Oxford University Press.

Brayne, C. and Ames, D. (1988). The epidemiology of mental disorders in old age. In *Mental Health Problems in Old Age*. (B. Gearing, M. Johnson and T. Heller, eds.) Chichester: Wiley.

Burn, W. and Drearden, T. (1990). Physical aspects of elderly depression, *Geriatr. Med.*, May, 61–64.

Burns, A., Jacoby, R. and Levy, R. (1990) Psychiatric phenomena in Alzheimer's disease. *Br. J. Psychiatry*, **157**, 72–94.

Burnside, I. M. (1988). *Nursing and the aged: a self care approach*. USA: McGraw-Hill.

Conway, P. (1988). Losses and grief in old age. *J. Contemp. Soc. Work*, November, 541–549.

Department of Health (1991). *The Health of the Nation: Health Survey for England 1991*. London: HMSO.

Department of Health (1992a). *Health and Personal Social Services Statistics for England*, London: HMSO.

Department of Health (1992b). *Health of the Nation: a Strategy for Health in England*. London: HMSO.

Ebersole, P. and Hess, P. (1990). *Toward healthy aging: human needs and nursing response*. St Louis, MO: Mosby.

Farran, C. J. and Keane-Haggerty, E. (1989). Communicating effectively with dementia patients. *J. Psychosoc. Nurs.*, **27**(5), 13–16.

Friedland, R. P. (1992). Dementia. In *Oxford Textbook of Geriatric Medicine*. (J. G. Evans and T. F. Williams, eds.), pp. 483–489. Oxford: Oxford University Press.

Gambert, S. R. and Hartford, J. T. (1991). Alcoholism in old age. In *Principles and Practice of Geriatric Medicine*. (M. S. J. Pathy, ed.), pp. 221–227, Chichester: Wiley.

Garrett, G. (1992). Health screening for elderly people. *Nurs. Stand.*, **6**(40), 25–27.

Henderson, A. S. (1992). The epidemiology of mental disorders in elderly people. In *Oxford Textbook of Geriatric Medicine*. (J. G. Evans and T. F. Williams, eds.) pp. 617–620. Oxford: Oxford University Press.

Hildick-Smith, M. (1991). Parkinson's disease. In *Principles and Practice of Geriatric Medicine.* (M. S. J. Pathy, ed.) pp. 803–816. Chichester: Wiley.

Hogstel, M. O. Ed. (1990). *Geropsychiatric nursing*. St Louis, MO: Mosby.

Jolley, D. J. and Jolley, S. P. (1991). Psychiatry of the elderly. In *Principles and Practice of Geriatric Medicine*. (M. S. J. Pathy, ed.). pp. 895–932. Chichester: Wiley.

Kane, R. A. and Bayer, A. J. (1991). Assessment of functional status. In *Principles and Practice of Geriatric Medicine*. (M. S. J. Pathy, ed.). pp. 265–278. Chichester: Wiley.

Knopman, D. S. and Sawyer-DeMaris, S. (1990). Practical approach to managing behavioural problems in dementia patients. *Geriatrics*, **45**(4), 27–35.

Lindesay, J. (1993). Suicide in the elderly. *Geriatr. Med.*, **23**(6), 48–53.

Lipowski, Z. J. (1992). Delirium and impaired consciousness. In *Oxford Textbook of Geriatric Medicine*. (J. G. Evans and T. F. Williams, eds.). pp. 490–496. Oxford: Oxford University Press.

Livingston, G. (1994). Understanding dementia; the rarer dementias. *J. Dementia Care*, **2**(4) 27–29.

Marr, J. (1994). The impact of HIV on older people. *Nurs. Stand.*, **8**(46), 28–31.

Murphy, E. (1992). Concepts of depression in old age. In *Oxford Textbook of Geriatric Medicine*. (J. G. Evans and T. F. Williams, eds.). pp. 620–634. Oxford: Oxford University Press.

Nelson, M. K. (1990). Organic mental disorders. In *Geropsychiatric Nursing*. (M. O. Hogstel, ed.). St Louis, MO: Mosby.

Norman, I. J. (1991a). Confusional states and dementia. In *Nursing Elderly People*. (S. Redfern, ed,). pp. 309–340. London: Livingstone.

Norman, I. J. (1991b). Mental health problems of elderly people: assessment and planning. In *Nursing Elderly People*. (S. Redfern, ed.). pp. 289–308. London: Livingstone.

Office for National Statistics. (1994). *Soc. Trends*, 94. London: HMSO.

O'Riordan, T. et al. (1989). The prevalence of depression in an acute geriatric medical assessment unit. *Int. J. Geriatr. Psychiatry*, **4**, 17–21.

Rabins, P. V. (1992). Cognition. In *Oxford Textbook of Geriatric Medicine*. (J. G. Evans and T. F. Williams, eds.). pp. 479–483. Oxfrod: Oxford University Press.

Rabins, P. V., Merchant, A. and Nestadt, G. (1984). Criteria for diagnosing reversible dementia caused by depression. *Br. J. Psychiatry*, **144**, 488–492.

Riley, B. (1990). Schizophrenia, paranoid disorders, anxiety disorders and somatoform disorders. In *Geropsychiatric Nursing*. (M. O. Hogstel, ed.). St Louis, MO:

Mosby.

Tallis, R. (1992). Epilepsy. In *Oxford Textbook of Geriatric Medicine*. (J. G. Evans and T. F. Williams, eds.). pp. 537–546. Oxford: Oxford University Press.

Tobiansky, R. (1993). Understanding dementia: Alzheimer's disease. *J. Dementia Care*, **1**(1), 26–28.

Tobiansky, R. (1994a) Understanding dementia: vascular dementia. *J. Dementia Care*, **2**(2), 23–24.

Tobiansky, R. (1994b). Understanding dementia: diffuse lewy body disease. *J. Dementia Care*, **2**(3), 26–27.

Working Party on Care of the Dementing Elderly. (1988). *Health Bull.*, **46**(2), 127–137.

Yurick, A. G., Spier, B. E., Robb, S. S. and Ebert, N. J. (1989). *The Aged Person and the Nursing Process*. East Norwalk, CT: Appleton and Lange.

4

Developing therapeutic nursing relationships with older people

James Marr

Introduction

> The crucial determinant of whether nursing is therapeutic or not is the quality of the relationship between nurse and patient. The power of nursing to promote healing lies, we believe, in this therapeutic relationship.
>
> (Muetzel, 1988)

This chapter seeks to explore the relationships that develop between nurses and older people and how these may help, or hinder, recovery from illness. Since the 1980s, 'value for money' has been a major feature within the health-care system and there has been a focus on the value of trained nurses. Over the years, much literature has accumulated from research projects that have attempted to identify the value of the nurse–patient relationship and the therapeutic benefit that it brings.

The relationships that develop between nurses and older people will be examined in the text, and an attempt made to identify and clarify the therapeutic benefit that these may have, not only for the older person but also for the nurse. The special challenge presented by older people with mental health problems and of addressing their specific needs will be investigated.

Communicating and building relationships with this group of people appear to be major difficulties for some nurses and many freely admit that they cannot do this type of nursing. I will therefore seek to identify particular issues concerning why this may prove to be so difficult for some nurses, particularly in relation to this patient/client group. It is hoped, therefore, that some of the subtle skills will be identified and clarified, because older people with mental health problems will become more visible and feature in larger numbers in most areas of health care provision in the future.

Aim

This chapter will endeavour to identify and clarify the skills involved in forming and maintaining therapeutic nursing relationships with older people who have mental health problems. Most commonly, issues surrounding the care of individuals with depressive illness or with dementia appear to offer the greatest challenge for nursing staff and the author will therefore focus the text particularly on meeting these needs, although the skills involved in implementing and maintaining therapeutic nursing relationships are transferable and need only to be modified to suit individual needs.

Rationale/background

Keep young and beautiful
It's your duty to be beautiful.
Keep young and beautiful
If you want to be loved.

From the song by Dubin and Warren (1922)

Negative stereotypes of old age permeate modern society as everyone strives for youthfulness. The words of the song are, unfortunately, too accurate in describing modern-day attitudes, even though it was written many years ago. This negative view of later life is especially common when one considers mental health and the term 'senile' is frequently used when describing older people. It is perhaps most unfortunate that these views are also held by health care professionals; the negative terminology that is frequently used is a visible sign of underlying negative attitudes. Slater and Gearing (1988) illustrate these attitudes with a quote from Dr Samuel Johnson, written in the eighteenth century:

There is a wicked inclination in most people to suppose an old man decayed in his intellects. If a young or middle aged man, when leaving company, does not recollect where he has laid 'his hat, it is nothing; but if the same inattention is discovered in an old man, people will shrug their shoulders and say, 'his memory is going'.

Depressive illness is perhaps the most common mental disorder of older age groups, with prevalence estimates ranging from six to twelve per cent of those aged sixty-five years and over (Victor, 1991). It is argued that much of depression in later life is a response to life events and losses, such as bereavement, despite the fact that many psychologists look for a biological cause in the first instance.

The dementing illnesses have been widely researched. Prevalence studies produce rates of between 2.5% and 9.3% in those aged over sixty-five (Victor, 1991), thus rating them as the second most common mental health disorder in later life. Both of these sets of statistics may be questioned, however, because missed diagnosis and underreporting are common with each of the disorders, thus reducing the numbers diagnosed. What is clear, however, is that with increasing age, the incidence of both types of illness also increases. With the projected demographical trends of the UK's ageing population, the challenges presented to the health care system will be even greater than that faced today. With the move towards care in the community, this challenge will be met by informal care networks as well as by professionals. Nurses are therefore in an ideal position to demonstrate their skill in this area and to educate others.

Literature review

As previously mentioned, there is a wealth of research and published material on the nurse–patient relationship. This has been carried out in various settings and with different grades of nursing staff and types of patients.

A review of psychiatric nursing textbooks over the years highlights the perceived value of nurses and the special therapeutic skills that they bring to patient care. Ironbar (1983) states that the nurse–patient relationship 'involves the establishment of an early rapport with the patient and his family'. The characteristics of the relationship are described thus:

- Trust
- Tolerance
- Understanding
- Warmth
- Friendliness
- A sympathetic sense of humour
- Acceptance
- Empathy

Earlier attempts to define mental health nursing and nursing skills are described by Peplau (1952) as 'a significant therapeutic, interpersonal process . . . that aims to promote forward movement of personality in the direction of creative, constructive, productive, personal and community living'.

Similarly, Travelbee (1964) claims nursing is an 'interpersonal process whereby the professional nurse practitioner assists an individual, family or community to prevent or cope with the experience of illness and suffering and, if necessary, to find meaning in these experiences'.

Salvage (1990), however, disagrees with these notions for general hospital patients, claiming that they do not necessarily want a close relationship with the nurse: 'The immediate concern is likely to be relief from pain and discomfort, rather than a meaningful relationship.' She does, however, stress the need for all to be treated with warmth, kindness and sensitivity. Perhaps in most 'general' areas, patients do not stay long enough for a meaningful relationship to develop, as all such relationships require an investment of time and the characteristics outlined above by Ironbar cannot be demonstrated effectively over a few days.

In a study of 'caring', McKenna (1993) appears to support the claims made by Salvage. She states that: 'Nurses appear to consider trusting and comforting types of behaviour most important, while patients favour behaviours associated with competency and physical care.'

These notions, however, are not widely accepted by others. Muetzel (1988) places great therapeutic value on the relationship between nurse and patient. In an attempt to describe this, she breaks the relationship into three components which overlap each other. These components are identified as 'intimacy', 'partnership' and 'reciprocity'. Intimacy and partnership together make up the 'atmosphere' of the relationship and forge the 'attitudes' that nurses have, while partnership and reciprocity produce the 'dynamics' of the encounter, which affect the things nurses do. Reciprocity and intimacy together give the 'spirit' of the relationship which determines how the nurse and patient 'are' together. In this way, a holistic therapeutic relationship is formulated.

Morse (1991) claims that one of four types of relationship may develop between nurse and patient, depending on certain circumstances such as the duration of contact, the needs of the patient, the commitment of the nurse and other personality factors. The four types of relationship that may emerge are identified as 'clinical', 'therapeutic', 'connected' and 'overinvolved'. From a superficial clinical basis the relationship proceeds to the type on which the nurse and patient implicitly agree. Either party may be unwilling to develop the process and a unilateral relationship thus ensues, with negative behaviours emerging.

Clinical relationships are described as being brief, with little emotional or personal involvement. They last only for a short time, the patient being satisfied with the professional service given. *Therapeutic relationships* are defined as 'ideal' and are the most common. They are of short duration involving fairly routine physical and psychosocial needs, which are met by the nurse; the patient feels secure and confident in the nurse's abilities. A more meaningful relationship is described as *connected* when enough time is spent for it to evolve beyond clinical or therapeutic limits. A trust develops and the nurse will bend rules to meet the needs of the patient and will act as an advocate on his or her behalf, giving protection from the unpleasant aspects of nursing care. The patient recognizes that the nurse has done more than was asked and is grateful. The nurse feels satisfied and fulfilled. The relationship is special and is remembered by both parties. The fourth type of relationship is even more intense and is described as *overinvolved*. This relationship develops beyond professional boundaries and becomes personal. Often the nurse becomes territorial about providing care to the patient, thus losing objectivity, and commitment shifts from others to the individual patient. Even after discharge, the nurse remains influential in a relationship based on mutual respect, care and trust which is often at the expense of his or her professional reputation.

The basis of nurse–patient relationships stems from the concept of 'therapeutic use of self', which originated in the field of psychotherapy. This concept recognizes the benefit of continued interpersonal interactions between the therapist and the client, which encourage support and help to change behaviour. Similar benefits are perceived between nurses and patients. This notion has been identified in recent years in the 'primary nursing' system of delivering care and, more recently, in the concept of the 'named nurse', in which the therapeutic value of the nurse–patient relationship is acknowledged and utilized.

Relationships with older people

I want to grow old comfortably,
life hanging on my shoulders
like an old sweater –
warm and loose and shapeless.

(Carmen Smith, 1994)

It is easy to forget that old age is a new experience for everyone and that with it come a host of adjustments, losses, disappointments, unmet needs and unachieved ambitions. We all hope and strive for a 'comfortable' old age but none of us knows what it will bring and how best to prepare ourselves for it. Fennell et al. (1989) describe the 'social construction of old age' in which older people are viewed as a social problem and a 'burden' to modern society. There is no doubt that many older people are generally a socially underprivileged group, due to poor finances, housing and health, and to loneliness, and that the effects of these and other stressors may affect their coping mechanisms. This in turn can affect their ability to relate to and communicate with others and they may appear suspicious, unfriendly or stubborn, hanging on desperately to their last symbols of independence. The old values to which they cling may appear outdated and silly in the context of modern society and they may view offers of help as 'charity', which causes them offence.

It is important, therefore, to allow time for a relationship to develop. This may involve a certain amount of tolerance and acceptance on the nurse's part, not moving too quickly or expecting everything at once. In their rush to 'assess' patients, nurses often forget that the patient also assesses them and for an older person, this may take some time. It is important to the older person to place the nurse in a social context and they will often be interested to know details of the nurse's background, family life, etc. In this way, there is a sharing of initial information as the older person decides whether or not the nurse is a 'nice person' and whether or not they will 'get on' together. Following this, it is necessary to find out if the nurse is 'a good nurse' who is competent, reliable and trustworthy.

Much of this initial assessment is done on the appearance of the nurse and it is important to remember that older people may have fairly narrow perceptions of how a nurse should look or behave (see Marr and Matthews, 1993). The nurse's display of warmth, friendliness and sympathy will be assessed as much by nonverbal communication, such as facial expression, as by what is said. An overpatronizing manner or childlike treatment will be spotted quickly and resisted.

As the relationship develops, it is important that the older person feels that the nurse is interested in what is said. Active listening skills, with good eye contact, head nodding and reflection on the content of the dialogue, will therefore help to reinforce this as both move towards an understanding of each other. The nurse attempts to see the world as the older person does and the older person feels accepted and understood. These important attributes communicated by the nurse during the interaction are described by Ersser (1992) as 'presentation' and 'presence'. They are fundamental to the success of the relationship.

Building a therapeutic relationship with an older person may be further complicated by issues surrounding the process of ageing. A degree of sensory impairment, such as hearing or sight loss, may make communication extra difficult and the nurse must therefore be aware of this, making some attempt to assess the degree of impairment and using skills to overcome the loss as much as possible. In the first instance, this may involve the adjustment of body position or voice or using touch or gestures to aid communication. However, the use of aids for hearing or vision should not be overlooked because many older people may need encouragement to use them. Simple maintenance of aids such as adjustment or cleaning, may also be necessary to ensure their effectiveness.

The use of language may require consideration. Attempts should be made to speak clearly, in a concise, unambiguous fashion, as fatigue and unfamiliarity may hinder concentration in an older person. Occasionally it may be necessary to add gentle reminders of the point or direction of the conversation, especially if there is concentration difficulty or a degree of memory loss. Cultural differences, and even regional differences, can affect the use and interpretation of language, thus affecting the meaning.

Mental health of older people

When attempting to build relationships with older people, the nurse must also be aware of issues surrounding their mental health. Although some degree of mental frailty is not uncommon in this age group, it is important to remember that not all older people suffer from memory loss or confusion. Many cope very well in the face of adversity. Making this sort of presumption will almost certainly cause hurt and offence and will not encourage the development of relationships.

Sometimes, the effects of the stress facing older people in modern society reduces their coping skills, causing *distress*. This distress may manifest as apathy, poor concentration or forgetfulness and may thus result in some degree of mental health disturbance that cannot be described as a mental illness. At an initial interview, it is therefore important to make an attempt to assess and to separate distress from disease.

In a study carried out by Murphy in 1982, it was found that depressed older people had experienced significantly more severe life events, major social difficulties and poor physical health in the preceding year than had a control group. A wide range of causes was identified but it was the impact of the meaning of these events on the older persons' lives that concerned Murphy. These causes she identified as the 'significant stressors' of old age and found that they could be grouped under four headings: loss, attack, restraint and threat.

Losses are self-explanatory, with 'attack' being described as any external force that produces discomfort, injury or pain. Restraints may similarly be due to external forces that restrict the actions necessary to meet basic needs or drives, these being reduced stamina, finances, sensory perception, or failing health. However, restraint may also be imposed by rules, regulations and other similar restrictions. Worries about the future may be focused around perceived loss, attack or restraint as circumstances change and the person feels more vulnerable. These are defined as 'threats' and centre around abandonment, disability, suffering or death.

Although these may represent very real fears for older people, it is important to remember that many cope extremely well in the face of adversity. Blazer (1982) attributes these coping skills to continued social interaction and the perceived social support from others. Murphy upholds this notion from her own work, demonstrating the importance of having an intimate confidante as a protection from stress and in maintaining good morale and good mental health. In her study, the value of this confidante did not appear to be about the *quantity* of the interactions (i.e. the number of times they were together), but the *quality* of the interactions (i.e. mutual feelings of warmth, trust and acceptance, based on reciprocity).

This further highlights the importance of interpersonal relationships in the promotion of psychological wellbeing and as a protection from ill health. Thus, when considering the mental health needs of older people, the nurse–patient relationship may offer considerable therapeutic benefit, even if the interaction is only on an intermittent basis, such as community nurse visits. It is the *quality* of time spent with the older person that matters for their well-being.

Nursing skills

To ensure this quality time within a relationship, the nurse must be very active, using communication and interpersonal skills to the full. This 'activity' is often described as the 'effective use of self' and is the basis of psychiatric nursing. The nurse attempts to view the world as the patient views it and to identify the personal beliefs and values of the individual. Burnard (1987) lists the particular skills required to do this:

- The ability to listen
- The ability to offer free attention
- The ability to suspend judgement
- The ability to offer accurate empathy

Listening must be an active process, requiring careful attention and concentration to hear properly what the other person is saying. It is vital to hear not only the words being used (i.e. the content) but to note the style or form of speech (i.e. volume, speed, structure and pitch). The observation of nonverbal communication (eye contact, movements, gestures, etc.) is also important to understand fully what is being said. A patient who is withdrawn and uncommunicative can really challenge the skills of the nurse. Similarly, an older person may not use language in the same way as the nurse, or may have some degree of sensory loss or cognitive impairment, maybe causing the nurse some real difficulty in understanding or following the conversation. Situations like this can be tiring for the nurse and for the patient and so it is important not to try to achieve too much at once but rather to attempt to have shorter, more frequent times together. *Attention* can therefore be difficult, especially if the nurse is working hard to accept and to take note of what is being said, encouraging the older person to express him or herself freely, without *judgement*. In listening actively, attempting to understand and to learn how the person perceives the world and him or herself, the nurse in turn offers, or tries to offer, *empathy*. If this feeling is not communicated or perceived as genuine, the relationship is inhibited. For the inexperienced nurse, the older person may often be difficult to convince!

This commitment and perseverance required of the nurse in attempting to build a therapeutic relationship is described by Pam Smith (1992) as 'emotional labour'. It is often a very demanding part of a nurse's work. Caring for, and caring about, others requires emotional effort and may be as hard as physical or technical labour. An older person who is suffering from a depressive or dementing illness may tax all of the nurse's skills of patience and dedication, even after only a short time. In situations like this, care is best carried out by more than one nurse, so that time is shared and some degree of relief and support is available to the nurses. Perhaps this emotional fatigue is why many nurses shy away from this type of work.

Qualities of the nurse

Nursing staff who succeed in caring for older people with mental health problems may thus possess extra skills, talents or qualities to which their success can be attributed. In addition to the characteristics identified by Ironbar earlier in the text, I would suggest that these nurses have also achieved a level of self-awareness and maturity that enables them to be philosophical about their work, identifying priorities from a wider viewpoint and perhaps being content with an inner feeling of job satisfaction rather than with obvious external rewards. In the work role they are flexible and adaptable with a commonsense, but creative, ability to problem-solve, carrying out their duties with composure and confidence, being clear about their responsibilities surrounding risk-taking and accountability. As far as possible, family and relatives are encouraged to be partners in care, with the patient's rights and choice always being the main consideration in the decisions made. Thus, this is not the job for the nurse who seeks power, order and control!

How many of the qualities of the nurse are therefore intrinsic and part of his or her character and how many are learned or acquired through experience? This is obviously difficult to say. Certainly, an interest in older people and their welfare would seem to be a necessity, as would the communication and interpersonal skills detailed. However, the registered nurse must also possess a sound knowledge of the physical and mental health problems that commonly affect older people and the effects of the ageing process on the presentation and management of these conditions. As explained throughout this book, physical and mental health are closely related in older people, in whom they are strongly influenced by psychosocial needs and their own perceived role in society. In any situation involving the provision of care and/or support, all of these factors must be considered and taken into account. Very often, they are finely balanced and this equilibrium is so easily upset by well-meaning health or social services personnel. If circumstances become unstable, the older person can quickly be catapulted into the orbit of the 'caring' professions, where their rights, freedom, choice and independence are threatened and they become victims of the very services that are set up to protect them.

Conclusion

As with other age groups, in older people the development and encouragement of close relationships with others is an important part of human existence. In the absence of effective, meaningful communication within a close relationship, people lose the opportunity to learn what effect they are having on others. This lack of positive self-appraisal and the lack of supportive feedback may cause self-esteem to suffer. When adequate support is available, coping mechanisms are strengthened and strategies to reduce stressful life circumstances come into play. It is the quality of time invested in these relationships that is more important than the quantity of time spent.

The special relationship that develops between nurses and patients may therefore be extremely therapeutic – more so than any medical treatment that is offered – and, for older people, this may be a lifeline while they strive to cope with changes and losses in later life. For those older people who have mental health problems, the nurse may be perceived as the only person who listens and attempts to understand their predicament, and it may be that nurse who gives insight and meaning, helping them pull the pieces together when the rest of their life is fragmenting.

It is in this kind of situation that the knowledge, skills and value of the nurse are most effectively demonstrated. However, these may remain unrecognized and unacknowledged by anyone but the patient; thus, the therapeutic benefit may never be fully explained or expressed.

References

Blazer, D. (1982). *Depression in Late Life*. St Louis, MO: Mosby.

Burnard, P. (1987). Sharing a viewpoint. *Senior Nurse*, **7**(3), 39.

Dubin, A. and Warren, H. (1922). *Keep Young and Beautiful*. London: Feldman/EMI Music.

Ersser, S. (1992). A search for the therapeutic dimensions of nurse–patient interaction. In *Nursing As Therapy*. (R. McMahon and A. Pearson, eds.). pp. 43–84, London: Chapman and Hall.

Fennell, G., Phillipson, C. and Evers, H. (1991). *The Sociology of Old Age*. pp. 52–59, London: Open University Press.

Ironbar, N. (1983). *Self-instruction in psychiatric nursing*. p. 8, London: Baillière Tindall.

Marr, J. and Matthews, T. (1993). Change of a dress. Nurs. Stand., **7**(19), 48–49.

McKenna, G. (1993) Caring is the essence of nursing practice. Br. J. Nurs., **2**, 72–76.

Morse, J. (1991). Negotiating commitment and involvement in the nurse–patient relationship. *J. Adv. Nurs.*, **16**, 445–468.

Muetzel, P. (1988). Therapeutic Nursing. In *Primary Nursing*. (A. Pearson, ed.), pp. 89–116. Kent: Croom Helm.

Murphy, E. (1982). Social origins of depression in old age. *Br. J. Psychiatry*, **141**, 135.

Peplau, H. (1952). *Interpersonal Relations in Nursing*. New York: Putnam.

Salvage, J. (1990). The theory and practice of the new nursing. *Nurs. Times*, **84**(4), 42–45.

Slater, R. and Gearing, B. (1988). Attitudes, stereotypes and prejudice about ageing', In *Mental Health Problems in Old Age* (B. Gearing, M. Johnson and T. Heller, eds.), p. 29. Milton Keynes: Open University.

Smith, C. (1994). Prayer for later days. In *On the Way Home*. (F. Makower and J. Faber, eds.). p. 33. London: Darton, Longman and Todd.

Smith, P. (1992). *Emotional Labour of Nursing*. Basingstoke: Macmillan.

Travelbee, J. (1964). What's wrong with sympathy?. *Am. J. Nurs.*, **64**(1), 68–71.

Victor, C. (1991). Health and Health Care in Later Life. pp. 76–93, Buckingham: Open University Press.

5

Supporting the carers of older poeple with mental health needs

Maria Scurfield

Introduction

The need to support carers in the community has been recognized by many reports, including the Griffiths Report (1988), the Community Care Act (Department of Health, 1990), the Carers Act (Department of Health, 1995). However, persistent failure to understand the needs of carers adequately has precluded effective interventions by professionals. This chapter will promote the idea that nurses are in a pivotal position to provide care to both older people with mental health needs and their carers. Caregiving is a significant issue for nurses practising in a variety of health care settings and they must make a commitment to treat carers as valued partners.

The main issues explored in this chapter include research of the positive and negative experiences on caregiving and the 'cost' of such experiences to carers. A review of the implementation of the assessment and care management arrangements of the Community Care Act (Department of Health, 1990) will also be examined from the point of view of the carer. The self-identified needs of carers will be discussed and suggestions of good practice interventions that meet the needs of carers will be explored.

This chapter aims to prov de the reader with a greater understanding of the caregiving experience, thereby providing insight into a range of nursing interventions that will meet the complex and changing needs of carers.

Learning outcomes

At the end of this chapter the reader will be able to:

1. Identify the number of informal carers in the UK

2. Describe six types of behaviour of a person suffering from dementia that may have a negative impact on the sufferer and the carer
3. List the four main areas that prove to be 'costs' to carers
4. Identify four major deficiencies and areas of need in carers interventions with professionals
5. Suggest nursing interventions that would meet the needs of carers

Rationale/background

The development of community care policies in the UK leaves carers with critical responsibilities. Since the late 1980s, there have been important demographic changes in society. People now live longer and the longer they live the more at risk they are from chronic ailments that impair their ability to care for themselves. Despite health problems, people survive for longer periods of time because of medical advances. The increase in the number of older people who need care coincides with a decrease in the number of family members who are able to care for them.

Factors that direct this unequal balance of supply and demand are: that people now live longer; the decreasing number of children per family; the reduction in the number of three-generation families that share joint households; a wider geographical distribution of family members; and a development towards equal opportunities for men and women as a result of which more women are employed in the labour force (Duijnstee, 1992). The change in family roles suggests that our generation will not accept caring responsibilities without an increase of resources.

Yet, despite these facts, there has been an explosion in caregiving research, which indicates that most families are committed to caring for dependent relatives at home, and many families continue to keep relatives at home even when they themselves are suffering extreme levels of stress (Braithwaite, 1990). Along with the rising tide of the older population comes the fact that more people will develop dementia. It is currently estimated that there are 636 000 people with dementia in the UK; this includes approximately 17 000 people with young-onset dementia. By the year 2021 it is estimated that this figure will rise to approximately 894 000 (Alzheimer's Disease Society, 1995).

The Government's philosophy of maintaining dependency groups in the community, coupled with the rising numbers of older people in the population, the reduction in NHS continuing care beds, and a dwindling pool of informal carers, highlights the need for appropriate professional intervention in this area. There has been a failure in the past of health care workers to understand fully the needs of family caregivers. This has resulted in interventions often being inappropriate, irrelevant or unavailable (Nolan and Grant, 1989; Twigg and Atkin, 1994).

The challenge to nurses is to become more aware of the family caregiving experience, to identify carers in their own working areas, and consider how they can best assess, and then plan, to meet their needs. Nurses must help carers to assess the difficulties and the satisfactions of their caregiving roles. This enables both the carer and nurse to explore alternative coping strategies that will enhance the caregiving/receiving experience.

Care packages designed to meet both the needs of the older person with mental health needs and the needs of the carer can have a major impact on increasing the quality of life of both parties.

Literature review

The informal carers

The 1990 General Household Survey (Office of Population Censuses and Surveys, 1992) suggests that at any one time 6.8 million people have caring responsibilities. One adult in seven (fourteen per cent) in the UK provides informal care and one in five households contains a carer. Between 1985 and 1990 the proportion of carers, whose main dependant was aged eighty-five years or over, increased from fifteen per cent to twenty per cent, and more than half had dependants who were aged seventy-five years or over. In 1990, as in 1985, more than two-thirds of carers were looking after female dependants. A total of 2.9 million carers are men and 3.9 million are women (Office of Population Censuses and Surveys, 1992). Around one million people provide care at home for thirty-five hours or more each week, and twenty per cent of carers look after more than one person. Carers come from all social groups and educational backgrounds. All age groups from youth to old age are represented; fifty per cent of carers are over pensionable age (Parker and Lawton, 1994).

The experience of caregiving

A review of the literature indicates that the toll of caregiving can be very high. For some carers, care may be satisfying and a source of companionship; for others it may prove an exhausting, frustrating and a seemingly endless commitment.

Under some circumstances, caregiving is transformed from the ordinary exchange of assistance to an extraordinary and unequally distributed burden. The emergence of a prolonged and serious impairment, such as dementia, is such a circumstance. A profound change in relationships occurs when impairment leads to increasing dependency on others for the satisfaction of basic needs (Pearlin et al., 1990).

Carers of dependants who are suffering from dementia are the hidden victims of the disease. Studies relating to dementia suggest that repetitive behaviours, inappropriate levels of activity, suspicious and destructive behaviours, sleep disturbances, wandering, incontinence, poor mobility and an inability to carry out personal care, such as dressing and bathing, are most troublesome symptoms for both sufferers and carers (George and Gwyther, 1986; O'Connor et al., 1990; Chappell and Penning, 1996). Cognitive deterioration can cause imbalance in a relationship. The dramatic and involuntary alteration of a cherished relationship is itself a major source of stress (Pearlin, 1983; Bass et al., 1994). Indeed, an overview of the research literature suggests that the symptoms of the dementia in relation to the deterioration of caregivers' wellbeing are overridden by fear for the future, which has been reported frequently as the problem that erodes caregiver management, ability and morale, and increases strain and tension (Zarit et al., 1980; Wilson, 1989).

This stress can be extreme. Studies of carers have found a high prevalence of psychiatric diagnoses (Gilleard et al., 1984; Schulz et al., 1993). Despite this, carers often wish their caring role to continue with support and help, and the decision to resort to institutional care is often only as a result of a lack of resources at home.

Caring costs

A further review of the relevant literature suggests that there are four main areas that will prove to be 'costs' to carers in the maintenance of their caring role. These include employment and financial costs, social costs, emotional and psychological costs, and physical costs (Allen, 1983; Butterworth, 1995; Woods, 1995).

Financial costs involve the direct extra expenses that arise because there is a dependant living in the household. This can include items such as extra heating, laundry, clothing, special diets and transport. Carers may also have to give up a job, or move to part-time work.

Social costs occur when there may be increasing isolation and disruption to normal life styles. Carers who are unable to leave their dependants alone safely can become confined to the house.

Stress and distress may be caused by providing continual care, often without respite, to dependants who are undergoing changes in their personality. Physical costs can occur as a result of problems with lifting, bathing and washing. Care is often provided by spouses who are usually elderly themselves and who also may have physical illnesses. Sleepless nights and having to be on hand twenty-four hours a day to prevent accidents takes its toll on carers' physical wellbeing.

Carers' needs

Caring builds up slowly. There is rarely a conscious decision or evidence of forward planning. Therefore, carers can feel taken for granted by their dependants, other family members, the public and professionals. Carers often have no training and are unprepared for the role reversals and responsibilities that are a consequence of caring. Their lack of recognition may cause anger and carers' needs may be ignored in preference to the dependant. There is a remarkable consensus on the help that carers want from professional service providers. Nolan and Grant (1989) identify four common areas of self-identified needs by carers: information, skills training, emotional support, and respite.

The implementation of the assessment and care management arrangements of the Community Care Act offers a positive step forward with the opportunity to provide a more flexible needs-led service.

Two reports indicate that there is still a long way to go to improve services for carers. *Deprivation and Dementia*, a report by the Alzheimer's Disease Society (1993) produced some alarming findings from the 1303 carers who were surveyed:

- Forty-two per cent of carers stated that they needed more professional help or respite care.
- Ninety-seven per cent of all carers were suffering from some form of emotional difficulty: stress (seventy per cent), tiredness (sixty-six per cent), depression (forty per cent) and loneliness (thirty-six per cent). Over a third of all carers surveyed (thirty-six per cent) have suffered from some form of physical problem as a direct result of being a carer.
- Twenty per cent of carers aged over eighty years were spending more than £300 a month on funding care.

The Carers' National Association report, *Community Care: Just a Fairytale?* (Warner, 1994) examined the effect of the implementation of the first year of the Community Care Act from the point of view of carers. Findings from the report revealed:

- Eighty per cent of carers agreed with the statement that community care changes made no difference to them.
- Twenty-seven per cent had not heard of community care.
- Seventy-four per cent of the carers surveyed had not received an assessment.

The Carers (Recognition and Services) Act 1995 came into effect in April 1996. Under the Act, local authorities are legally obliged to assess the ability of carers to provide and continue to provide care. The Act is targeted at an estimated 1.5 million carers who provide care for more than twenty or more hours a week (Arksey, 1996). It does not entitle carers to any services, but only gives them the right to an assessment. Carers' assessment is extremely important because in many cases, all a carer seeks is some form of recognition (Clements, 1996).

Carers require their views and ability to cope to be taken into account when a disabled person's care package is being devised, on the basis that the less able a carer is to cope, the more intensive the provision of service should be.

The NHS Community Care Act 1990 and the Carers Act 1995 acknowledge carers as the major providers of community care. The Carers Act should result in improved statutory support for carers. However, it remains difficult to ascertain how much existing and new resources will be given to help to support carers.

Nursing interventions

The four major deficiencies and areas of need in carers' interactions with professionals include: lack of information; lack of skills; lack of emotional support and lack of sufficient respite. These areas provide a useful organizing framework for nurses and other health care workers who are aiming to develop good practice with carers. Each area will be examined and suggestions of interventions that nurses can explore with the carers will be made.

Information

Studies indicate that carers do not have the time or the energy to search for information. The provision of information to carers is, however, crucial, as it can increase their sense of control over a caring situation and allow for a degree of informed choice.

Nurses need to be aware of locality-based services and what they provide in terms of help and support to carers. It is also necessary to be aware of referral patterns to such services, as it would only add to carers' stress to be told of a service, only to find their hopes dashed if the service had a waiting list, or no longer exists.

The provision of a resource corner in your work location, containing a wide range of information that carers could use would be very practical. Liaising with local statutory and voluntary agencies such as Social Services, community centres, advice centres, health information centres, libraries, Help the Aged, Age Concern, health promotion, Family Health Services Association etc., would be a starting point for building up resources. There are many national organizations that provide enormous amounts of information and support for carers. Apart from the very specific organizations such as the Alzheimer's Disease Society, there are also more general organizations, such as the Carers' National Association, Counsel and Care of the Elderly, Help the Aged, MIND etc.

It can be argued that nurses should not be responsible for updating such information because it entails enormous time constraints. However, if nurses and other health care workers are serious in their commitment to supporting carers, then it is necessary to be aware of relevant information that could help carers. Keady and Nolan (1994) suggest that providing information regarding dementia for the carer is indeed an integral part of good practice.

Nurses are also asked by carers to provide financial advice. They could help carers more by giving them information about appropriate contact points such as local advice centres, Social Services and civic centres. Nurses can ensure that families are receiving all the welfare benefits to which they are entitled, including benefits that can be claimed by the disabled or elderly person, as well as by the carer.

Some carers may find it confusing when trying to choose relevant information. Nurses should be sensitive to carers' needs and help them to choose appropriately. Individual reports by Ellis (1993) and Warner (1994) identify the need for service users to have access to high quality consistent information about a range of topics. However, both reports highlight gaps in the provision and the quality of information supplied.

Nurses also need to be sensitive towards giving the carers information regarding their dependant's illness and treatment. There is little doubt that most carers want this information. It could be argued that lack of knowledge can itself be a stressor because it causes anxiety, fear and uncertainty about what the future holds; in other words the carer does not have control of the situation. Studies have shown that providing information to carers of people with dementia helps both the carer and the person with dementia to adjust to their new roles (Coyne, 1991; Keady and Nolan, 1995). Accurate information not only increases carers' understanding but also reduces inappropriate perceptions and hostile feelings towards their dependants. However, caution is needed, as some carers, for example, those caring for relatives with a form of dementia, do not want to acknowledge the fact that their relative will deteriorate. Alternatively, carers who do want this information may, for the first time, have to face the fact that their dependants are not going to recover, and, worse still, that they will deteriorate. Carers can become very distressed at such a time. The implications for nurses facing this situation is clear. Carers should be monitored and individual support and counselling offered where necessary.

Checklist for good practice
- Have a knowledge of local resources that may help older persons with mental health needs and their carers
- Have an awareness of referral patterns to community resources
- Provide a resource area offering up-to-date information to carers in your work setting
- Provide information about national organizations to carers
- Have a sensitive approach when imparting information regarding a dependant's illness and treatment to a carer
- Provide a structured, personalized approach to the provision of information to carers

Skills training

Many carers who experience difficulty in coping do not admit this and avoid asking for help, which, in turn, leads to resource exhaustion. Many carers use up their own personal resources so that it is the breakdown of care that eventually receives attention in the last resort (Allen, 1983).

If community care is to be a success, then increased attention should be given to the area of skills training and self-care. It is vital to involve carers in self-care activities, both to assist their dependants and to enhance their own self-care strategies. It is significant that the reasons why carers often give up their role is because the dependant develops behavioural problems, becomes incontinent or is disruptive at night, thereby reducing the carer's quality of life.

Nurses can do much to help carers to develop coping strategies by adopting a sensitive approach towards them. Carers should be encouraged to discuss things that they find difficult in their caring role.

Nurses can encourage carers to explore a range of different strategies to enable them to cope with the difficulties, thereby enhancing both their quality of life and that of the older persons for whom they care. Carers should be advised to deal with day-to-day dilemmas using a problem-solving approach. For example, by dealing with one problem at a time, listing the advantages and disadvantages of interventions, listing ways to overcome the problem, and noting the outcome and effect of the interventions. This enables carers to have much more control over the situation.

If nurses could assist carers to find ways of managing difficult behaviours we would reduce positively the amount of stress that they experienced.

It may be necessary to refer the client or the carer to other members of the multidisciplinary team. For example, if the carer has difficulty in bathing their dependant relative, an occupational therapist and/or a physiotherapist may be the most appropriate member of the team to offer advice.

Checklist for good practice
- Encourage carers to discuss difficulties in the caregiving role
- Explore different coping strategies that may benefit the carer
- Encourage carers to adopt a problem-solving approach to dilemmas
- The various roles of the multidisciplinary team need to be clearly stated in terms that are easily understood by carers.

Emotional support

Studies indicate that the objective circumstances of caring contribute only in a small part to carer stress and that emotional elements are more significant. The published literature also indicates that it is apparent that carers are sensitive to the reactions of professionals and that poor reactions of professionals can not only increase carer stress levels but also inhibit carers from seeking further professional help. The results of a national carers' study (Nolan and Grant, 1989) showed that one of the greatest problems identified by carers related to poor professional attitudes. An improved professional attitude towards carers has the potential not only to reduce carer stress levels but also, by acknowledging their contribution, to heighten the satisfaction of caring.

Nurses need to be able to empathize with carers as well as to assist them to recognize and deal with a range of emotions. Carers often voice feelings of isolation, guilt and anger, while lacking a confidant(e) with whom they can share those emotions. In situations where the dependant is perceived to be overly demanding and unappreciative, caring is made all the more difficult. There have been many studies that confirm high levels of stress and depression in the caregivers of dementia sufferers. There are numerous assessment scales that nurses can utilize to measure levels of stress or distress in carers, for example:

- The thirty-item General Hospital Questionnaire (Goldberg, 1978) gives an index of emotional distress and is a self-administered questionnaire
- The thirteen-item Strain Scale (Gilleard, 1984) has less emphasis on the problems and more on how the supporter reacts to them
- The thirty-four Problem Checklist (Gilleard, 1984) rates the problem status for the supporter of various deficits or disturbing behaviours displayed by the dependant
- The carer's Assessment of Difficulties Index (Nolan and Grant, 1992)

This list is not exhaustive and other screening methods could be utilized if they were deemed to be appropriate.

There are a number of overriding features to be considered when using formal assessment scales. First of all, the needs of the person being cared for are paramount and specific training is essential to ensure safe practice.

Nurses also need to be aware that carers are very individual in the way in which they cope and react to their caring role. Some carers cope extremely well while caring for dependants with severe physical and mental health needs, only requiring limited support from health care professionals. On the other hand, many carers find it extremely difficult to cope with any changes in their dependant's physical or mental health. Sometimes these carers can present as being very angry and hostile. Initially, nurses may find it difficult to establish a therapeutic relationship with them. Carers' anger, which is sometimes directed at nurses, is often due to the conflicting emotions they are experiencing in their caregiving role. It is vitally important for nurses to remain calm in such situations and to allow carers to ventilate their feelings in a safe environment. Nurses can reduce carers' stress by acknowledging their contribution, by giving attention to the emotional aspects of caring, and by assisting them to find meaning in their situation. Carers should be encouraged to explore the satisfactions of their caregiving role because all too often attention is focused on the negative aspects of care. Studies have explored the positive dimensions in providing home care to people with dementia. Carers can experience warmth, comfort and pleasure (Kinney and Stephens, 1989; Grant and Nolan, 1993; Cohen et al., 1994). A carers' satisfaction index has been developed, which attempts to redress the focus of carers' experience to encourage them to explore the positive outcomes of their caring role (Nolan and Grant, 1992).

Checklist for good practice:
- Have a sensitive approach when interacting with carers
- Help carers to recognize and deal with the emotions of caregiving
- Recognize that carers are individual in the way they respond to their caring role
- Encourage carers to explore satisfactions in their caring role

Carers' support groups

Carers' support groups can have a beneficial impact on carers. They provide opportunities for carers to exchange experiences and discuss the management of problems (Fuller et al., 1979); allow carers to express feelings of sorrow, guilt and anger (North, 1985); offer self-help; supply information and advice (William, 1987); and provide structural training for carers (Saddington, 1986).

Studies of carers' groups that have been formally evaluated have shown many positive results. A recent study (Sharp and Scurfield, 1991) reported that a carers' support group was successful in increasing carers' knowledge of their dependant's illness, increasing their ability to manage problems, and increasing carers' awareness of how to obtain advice. Other results indicate that most carers felt more confident and less anxious in their caring role, and that they valued the emotional support obtained from other carers.

There is much disagreement about the types and levels of support that are required by carers and what can be expected from hard-pressed services and professionals. It is the tension between the varied needs of carers and the ability or willingness of others to meet their requirements that confronts nurses and other health professionals daily.

It is clear that there are advantages for nurses, and other health care workers in setting up carers' groups. If groups are designed to incorporate interventions including information provision, skills learning and emotional support, then such a model would provide a clear match between a practice model and carers' identified deficits, and would do much to redress the current imbalance of practice.

Designing a carers' support group

Bearing in mind the diversity of carer need and restrictions on the movement of carers, it would be almost impossible to arrange set courses for carers that are appropriate and accessible to all. Clearly, it needs to be borne in mind that many carers may find it difficult to attend carers' groups because of their caring responsibilities at home. Consideration needs to be given to the provision of a sitting service, which could be at home or at the place of the support group. The carer group environment could be used as an ideal setting for carer training and support if the group consisted of people dealing with the same type of disability.

Although some carers' support groups have been designed to incorporate the universal needs of carers, nurses can make the programme more relevant to their particular group by asking carers what they want from the group. Alternatively, carers could be asked by means of a questionnaire to identify the problems that they have and indicate how stressful that problem is to them. The use of both qualitative and quantitative questions should make the information more relevant. A programme could then be designed to tackle the most common problems and needs that the carers have identified.

Questionnaires could also include items on the most relevant format for the group (for example, an informal group setting, an educative group or a mixture of both). If carers state that they need advice or training on different issues, then the nurse could invite appropriate guest speakers to the group. (For example, in dealing with continence, a continence adviser could be invited.) It would be advantageous to have one or two nurses (or health care professionals) to facilitate the group throughout the course of the programme. This would also help to identify any carers who need individual counselling.

It is recognized that there are problems with close involvement by professionals. They may have an inhibitive effect on members' freedom of expression. Becoming involved to the extent of acting as group representative/advocate in interactions with the statutory authorities could compromise a nurse's own position. However, it is also acknowledged that, in order to maximize the group's chances of survival and development, ongoing professional support will be necessary. It could, therefore, be advisable that professional involvement should gradually be withdrawn to the extent that they could be freely available for support and advice, while also giving the group optimum independence.

Checklist for good practice
- Design carers' group to incorporate interventions that include information, skills training and emotional support
- Ascertain what the carers want from the group before planning it
- Encourage the carers to evaluate the group formally; this evaluation will prove useful when organizing further carers' groups
- The various roles of the multidisciplinary team need to be clearly stated in terms that are easily understood by the carers

Respite

Carers need relief from their twenty-four-hour role. This may range from a few hours a day or an evening, to whole weeks when holidays can be taken. Respite may be provided by day centres, sitting services or purpose-built respite units. Respite can have a positive effect on carers' physical and emotional health. Nurses need to be aware of the availability of respite facilities in their own area and be able to offer this information to carers. Some carers express feelings of guilt and hopelessness about respite care for their dependant. It is extremely important that carers are treated sensitively when using respite services; they should not feel that they are abandoning their dependant or feel guilty for taking a break. Nurses could also encourage carers to help to develop for their dependant a care plan that is based on normal daily routines and specific aspects that they feel are important during the respite care.

Checklist for good practice
- Be sensitive to carers' feelings about accepting respite care
- Encourage carers to participate in planning the care of their dependants
- Ensure that the aspects of care that are deemed important by carers are facilitated

Summary

The philosophy of maintaining dependency groups in the community, along with the rising numbers of older people, has highlighted the need for appropriate interventions in this area.

At some point in our lives, most of us will either be unpaid carers or be cared for at home by relatives or friends. For some carers, such as those looking after someone with dementia, the job is a twenty-four-hour, 365-days-a-year commitment.

A greater understanding of the caregiving experience offers insight into appropriate practice interventions. Caregiver stress is not a universal occurrence. There are great differences in carers' circumstances, experiences and responses that have an impact on their ability to cope. As the dependant's needs change, so will those of the carers. The four areas of need identified by carers provide a useful framework for nurses to develop suitable practice models for carers.

Nurses need to foster an approach that offers carers emotional and educational support, thereby transferring the skills and knowledge they possess to sustain the commitment that is so apparent in carers. There is no doubt that carers wish to be treated as partners, and be valued and recognized for their role, and be consulted regarding the services they receive. Carers need to be viewed as true partners in care. The challenge with which nurses are faced is to develop flexible services at a pace that meets the complex, challenging and changing needs of carers.

References

Allen, I. (1983). *Elderly People in the Community: Their Service Needs*. London: HMSO.

Alzheimer's Disease Society. (1993). *Deprivation and Dementia*. London: ADS.

Alzheimer's Disease Society. (1995). *Right from the Start: Primary Health Care and Dementia*. London: ADS.

Arksey, H. (1996). Missed target. *Community Care*. (1113), 24–26

Bass, D. M., McClendon, M. J., Deimling, G. T. and Mukherjees, S. (1994). The influence of a diagnosed mental impairment on family caregiver strain. *J. Gerontol. (Soc. Sci.)*, **49**, 146–155.

Braithwaite. V. A. (1990). *Bound to Care*. London: Allen and Unwin.

Butterworth, M. (1995). Dementia: the caregiver's perspective. *J. Ment. Health*, **4**, 125–132.

Chappell, N. L. and Penning, M. (1996). Behavioural problems and distress among caregivers. *Ageing Soc.*, **16**(1), 57–73.

Clements, L. (1996). Real act of care. *Community Care*, (1111) 26–27

Cohen, C. A., Pushkar-Gold., Shulman, K. I. and Zucchero, C. A. (1994). Positive aspects in caregiving: an overlooked variable in research. *Can. J. Ageing*, **13**, 378–391

Coyne, A. C. (1991). Information and referral services; usage among caregivers for dementia patients. *Gerontologist*, **31**, 384–388.

Department of Health. (1990). NHS and Community Care Act. London: HMSO.

Department of Health. (1995) The Carers' (Recognition and Services) Act. London: HMSO.

Duijnstee, M. (1992). Caring for a demented family member at home. In *Caregiving in dementia: Research and Applications.* (G. Jones and B. M. L. Meisen, eds.). pp. 359–379, London: Routledge.

Ellis, K. (1993). *Squaring the Circle: User and Carer Participation in Needs Assessment.* York: Joseph Rowntree Foundation.

Fuller, J., Ward, E., Evans, A. et al. (1979). Dementia: supportive groups for relatives. *Br. Med. J.,* **1**, 684–685.

George, L. K. and Gwyther, L. P. (1986). Caregiver well-being: a multi-dimensional examination of family caregivers of demented adults. *Gerontologist,* **26**, 253–259.

Gilleard, C. J., Belford, H., Gilleard, E., Gledhill, K. and Whittick, J. E. (1984). Emotional distress amongst supporters of the elderly infirm. *Br. J. Psychiatr.,* **145**, 172–177.

Goldberg, D. P. (1978). *Manual for the General Health Questionnaire.* Windsor: NFER - Nelson.

Grant, G. and Nolan, M. R. (1993). Informal carers: sources and concomitants of satisfaction. *Health Soc. Care Community,* **1**, 147–159

Griffiths, R. (1988). *Community Care – Agenda for Action.* (A report to the Secretary of State for the Social Services). London: HMSO.

Keady, J. and Nolan, M. R. (1994). The carer-led assessment process (CLASP): a framework for the assessment of need in dementia caregivers. *J. Clin. Nurs.,* **3**, 103–108.

Keady, J. and Nolan, M. R. (1995) A stitch in time. Facilitating proactive interventions with dementia caregivers: the role of community practitioners. *J. Psychiatr. Ment. Health Nurs.,* **2**, 33–40.

Kinney, J. M. and Stephens, M. P. (1989). Hassles and uplifts of giving care to a family member with dementia. *Psychol. Ageing,* **4**, 402–408.

Nolan. M. R. and Grant, G. (1989). Addressing the needs of informal carers: A neglected area of nursing practice. *J. Adv. Nurs.,* **114**, 950–961

Nolan, M. R. and Grant, G. (1992). *Regular Respite: An Evaluation of a Hospital Rota Bed Scheme for Elderly People. Age Concern Institute of Gerontology Research Papers Series No. 6.* London: Ace Books.

North, S. (1985). Breaking point. *Nurs. Mirror,* **161**, 42–43

O'Connor, D.W., Pollitt, P. A., Roth, M. et al. (1990) Problems reported by relatives in a community study of dementia. *Br. J. Psychiatr.,* **156**, 835–841

Office of Population Censuses and Surveys. (1992). *General Household Survey: Carers in 1990.* London: HMSO.

Parker, G. and Lawton, D. (1994). *Different Types of Care, Different Types of Carer: Evidence from the General Household Survey.* (Social Policy Research Unit). London: HMSO.

Pearlin, L. I. (1983). Role strains and personal stress. *In: Psychosocial Stress: Trends in Theory and Research.* (H. B. Kaplan, ed.) New York: Academic Press.

Pearlin, L. I., Mullan, J. T., Semple, S. J. and Skaft, M. (1990). Caregiving and the stress process: an overview of concepts and their measures. *Gerontologist*, **30**, 583–594.

Saddington, N. (1986). Training the carers. *Nurs. Times*, **82**, 42–43.

Sharp, T. and Scurfield, M. (1991). Needs of the carer: all in a days' work. *Nurs. Times*, **87**(35), 24–27.

Schulz, R., Williamson, G. M., Morycz, R. and Beigel, D. E. (1993). Changes in depression among men and women caring for an Alzheimer's patient. In *Caregivers' Systems: Formal and Informal Helpers*. (S. H. Zarit, L. I. Pearlin and S. Warner, eds.), Hillside, NJ: Erlbaum.

Twigg, J. and Atkin, K. (1994). *Carers Perceived: Policy and Practice in Informal Care*. Milton Keynes: Open University Press.

Warner, N. (1994). *Community Care: Just a Fairytale?* London: Carers' National Association.

William, P. (1987). Family feeling. *Community Outlook*. (January), 7–10.

Wilson, H. S. (1989). Family caregivers: the experience of Alzheimer's disease. *Appl. Nurs. Res.*, **2**, 40–45

Woods, B. (1995). Dementia care: progress and prospects. *J. Ment. Health*, **4**, 115–124.

Zarit, S. H., Reever, K. E. and Bach-Peterson, J. (1980). Relatives of the impaired elderly: correlates of feelings of burden. *Gerontologist*, **20**, 649–655.

Further reading

Biegel, D. E., Sales, E. and Schulz, R. (1991). *Family Caregiving in Chronic Illness*. Newbury Park, CA: Sage.

Ellis, K, (1993). Squaring the Circle: *User and Carer Participation in Needs Assessment*. York: Joseph Rowntree Foundation.

Henwood, M., Jowell. T. and Wistow. G. (1991). *All Things Come to Those Who Wait: Causes and Consequences of the Community Care Delays*. London: King's Fund Institute..

Hettiaratchy, P. and Manthorpe, J. (1992). A carer's group for families of patients with dementia. In *Caregiving in Dementia: Research and Applications*. (G. Jones, and B. M. L. Meisen, eds.), pp. 419–434. London: Routledge.

House of Commons Social Services Committee: Community Care. (1990). *Fifth Report: Carers*. London: HMSO.

Mace, N. L. and Rabins, P. V. (1985). *The 36-hour day*. London: Hodder and Stoughton.

Marshall, M. (19??). *I Can't Place This at All: Working with People with Dementia and Their Carers*. Birmingham: Ventura Press.

Nolan, M. R., Grant, G., Cadlock, K. and Keady, J. (1994). *A Framework for Assessing the Needs of Family Carers: A Multi-disciplinary guide*. Newcastle under Lyme: BASE publications.

Parker, G. (1985). *With Due Care and Attention: A Review of the Research on Informal Care*. London: Family Policy Studies Centre.

Quereshi, H. and Walker, A. (1989). *The Caring Relationship: Elderly People and Their Families*. London: Macmillan.

Robinson. J. and Yee, L. (1991). *Focus on Carers: A Practical Guide to Planning and Delivering Community Care Services.* London: King's Fund.

Smith, G. C., Smith, M. F. and Toseland, R. W. (1991). Problems identified by family caregivers in counselling. *Gerontologist*, **31**, 15–22

Training

Bradford Dementia Group. (1995) Structured support for dementia carers: a Person-Centred Approach (training course). University of Bradford.

Useful contacts

Age Concern England, Astral House, 1268 London Road, London SW16 4ER.

Alzheimer's Disease Society, Gordon House, 10 Greencoat Place, London. SW1P 1PH. Tel: 0171 306 0606

Carers' National Association, 20/25 Glasshouse Yard, London EC1A 1JS. Tel: 0171 490 8818

Counsel and Care, Twyman House, 16 Bonny Street, London NW1 9PG. Tel: 0171 485 1566

Help the Aged, St James' Walk, London EC1R 0BE. Tel: 0171 253 0253

National Association of Citizen's Advice Bureaux, Myddelton House, 115–123 Pentonville Road, London N1 9LZ. Tel: 0171 833 2181

6

Acute Confusional States

Irene Schofield and Hazel Heath

Introduction

Acute confusional states (ACS) are the most common type of psychiatric manifestation found in general hospital wards; a significant number of older people are affected. Although recovery is the most common outcome and, in most cases, the condition resolves completely within four weeks (American Psychiatric Association, 1987), an ACS is a medical emergency. It can often be a prelude to death and, in a small number of cases (something like five per cent), it is followed by dementia.

It is important to distinguish between acute confusional states (usually described as delirium in the American literature) and other, more ongoing, mental impairments.

Confusion is a symptom, not a diagnosis

Acute confusional states characteristically have an abrupt onset. They are usually temporary and reversible once the cause has been treated. Early recognition and treatment of the underlying cause is crucial, and nurses have a key role in providing physical, psychological and environmental support (Wolanin and Phillips, 1981). In situations where this is not appreciated, it is unlikely that the patient will receive the correct diagnosis and treatment. In studies of nurses' ability to identify hospitalized patients with ACS, forty-three per cent (Lucas and Folstein, 1980) and seventy-two per cent (Palmateer and McCartney, 1985) failed to do so.

Beliefs about mental impairment

One of the myths underpinning common beliefs about ageing, is that 'senility', or permanent mental impairment, is an inevitable consequence of

growing old. Health care professionals, including nurses, are not exempt
from this view. The perception of later life as a time when mental impairment is inevitable can have dire consequences for the person who presents
with an acute confusional state. It may mean that health care professionals'
efforts are not directed towards accurate diagnosis, appropriate treatment
and management, which may result in increasing deterioration and subsequent death.

The perception of later life as a time when mental impairment is inevitable
also accounts for the lack of research interest in this very common phenomenon which, if undetected, can threaten quality of life and the life chances of
the older person. This is now beginning to change slowly, thanks to a small
group of American nurse researchers who are pushing forward the boundaries of knowledge in this area and, at the same time, making it more acceptable as a topic for further study.

Beliefs about confusion

'Appears confused' and, 'confused at times' are common descriptions of
older people who exhibit signs of disorientation or other seemingly
inappropriate behaviour, irrespective of whether the cause is reversible or
preventable. Conceptions of the term 'confusion' vary between nurses, doctors and those who have studied the phenomenon in some detail.

Wolanin (1973) examined both medical and nursing records in a nursing
home, to determine how the behaviour of confused older individuals was
documented by both groups. She found that the doctors focused on cognitive deficits, especially those that interfered with their ability to take a case
history or with attempts to reach a diagnosis. Common comments were
'poor memory', 'poor historian', 'cannot understand directions'.

The nurses, on the other hand, described antisocial behaviours such as
'hostile', or 'difficult to manage'. Later, when interviewed in a more relaxed
atmosphere and when they were less inhibited, nurses resorted to such terms
as 'zombie', 'packrat' and 'screamer'.

'Pleasantly confused' is another relatively common description of behaviour, but it must be questioned whether there could really be anything pleasant about not being fully in touch with reality, or whether this is another
example of nurses perceiving the behaviour (whatever it is) as socially acceptable because it does not disrupt the scheme of work.

Both nurses and medical staff appeared to perceive the confused person as
someone who interfered with their ability to carry out their professional

responsibilities, rather than as an individual with complex needs. This view sits uncomfortably beside the notion of patient-centred care, which would have the patient's ability to function as its central concern, rather than his or her effect on the nurses. The perception of the acutely confused person in terms of being a nuisance will be revisited in the section on management.

Definitions of acute confusional state

According to Raisin (1990), nurses use 'confusion' as an all-encompassing term to describe the collection of cognitive and behavioural characteristics that accompany the medical diagnoses of dementia and ACS. First, it is important that nurses should link the 'confusion' with the correct diagnosis (i.e. ACS (reversible) or dementia (irreversible)). Secondly, nurses must be more precise in their identification and description of these characteristics, because they are diverse and require different methods of management. Not every characteristic will be present in all affected persons and, because of this, ACS is said to be idiosyncratic. Furthermore, recently-published work, cited by Foreman (1993), suggests that manifestations of particular characteristics are a function of the underlying cause of the ACS.

The variety of causes and manifestations of ACS make it a very complex phenomenon and, as one might expect, there is no single neat definition that covers all the aspects. Brooking (1986) defines acute or toxic confusion, or delirium, as 'an acute or subacute alteration in previously normal mental function, which is often temporary and reversible, associated with impaired brain function usually secondary to a pathological process outside the nervous system' (p. 242). Brooking's definition is useful in that it describes the effects of pathology as additional stressors to body systems, which are themselves affected by age-related decline. It also includes the transience of the phenomenon. It has the disadvantage, however, of not describing how ACS affects the individual in an observable way.

In order to research into the usefulness of a variety of preventive and ameliorative measures, Williams et al. (1985) provided the following behavioural definition:

> The verbal or non-verbal manifestations of disorientation to time, place, or persons in the environment; inappropriate communication or communication unusual for the person such as nonsensical speech, calling out, yelling, swearing, or unusual silence; inappropriate behaviour such as attempting to get out of bed, pulling at tubes, dressings, or picking at bedclothes; and illusions or hallucinations.

It is noteworthy that cognitive dimensions, such as poor memory and loss of attention and concentration, are not included in their definition.

Another commonly used definition is that provided by the American Psychiatric Association (1987): 'An acute confusional state is a simultaneous disturbance in consciousness, attention, perception, memory, thinking, orientation, psychomotor behaviour, and the sleep-wake cycle that develops abruptly and fluctuates diurnally.' This definition includes both cognitive and behavioural characteristics.

Practising nurses commonly cite alteration in level of orientation and alertness as being diagnostic of ACS. However, Foreman (1991) suggests that, in order to reach a definitive diagnosis of ACS, deficits in five areas must be observed. These are: cognition, orientation, motor behaviour, memory and higher integrative functions (judgement, hearing, cooperation and ability to perform some activities of daily living skills). He points out that the unfamiliar routines of a hospital stay can affect the circadian rhythms of those who are not diagnosed with ACS, causing them to experience some disorientation. Also, the level of motor activity might be governed by the cause of the ACS. For example, hyperactivity might be the result of cerebral hypoxia. Foreman also argues that deficits in cognitive characteristics, such as concentration and attention, are more sensitive indicators. He defines ACS as a 'transient state of cognitive impairment... a syndrome manifested by simultaneous disturbances of consciousness, attention, perception, memory, thinking, orientation, and psychomotor behaviour [that] develop abruptly, and fluctuate diurnally' (Foreman, 1991).

Causes of acute confusional state

Acute confusional states can occur at any age. However, they are most likely to be seen in the very young, when the central nervous system is in the process of maturation, or in the very old, when the ability to maintain homeostasis is affected by age-related changes in all body systems. Often, the ACS is the only indication of physical illness.

The phenomenon of altered presentation of disease is one of the essential differences between younger and older adults. In situations where this is not appreciated, it is unlikely that the patient will receive the correct diagnosis and treatment.

Brooking's definition, cited earlier, clearly outlines the essential cause of ACS. Its basic premise is that, for those people who develop ACS, cerebral functioning is already compromised by age-related changes, although, under the conditions of low physiological stress, cognitive function remains normal. However, the appearance of a systemic illness or physiological imbalance can disturb the delicate balance of cerebral metabolism, thus producing a significant impact on cognitive functioning. A reduction in cerebral metabolism decreases neurotransmitters in the brain, especially acetylcholine and adrenaline. Acetylcholine is essential for attention, learning, memory and information processing. The frontal and temporal lobes are most commonly affected. The brain therefore acts as a sensitive indicator of an underlying disease process. It monitors the general functioning of the body, so that disturbances of cognitive function signal the presence of systemic illness affecting other more distant body systems.

Foreman (1993) suggests that ACS has multiple rather than single causes, and that these represent all aspects of human illness and, in some cases, their treatment. Medications (especially anticholinergics and those affecting the central nervous system), infections (urinary tract and chest infection), electrolyte imbalances and metabolic disturbances, are generally cited as being the main causes of ACS.

Who is affected by acute confusional states, and what are the outcomes?

Those aged over sixty years are most at risk of developing ACS. The risk increases with age, and those aged eighty and over are most vulnerable. Between one-third and one-half of hospitalized older patients are likely to develop ACS at some point during their admission (Lipowski, 1983). Bearing in mind that the number of people aged eighty-five and over has increased by fifty per cent in the ten years from 1981 to 1991, and that the majority of health service users are older people, it is likely that there will be a corresponding increase in the incidence of older people who present with ACS. It is important, therefore, for nurses to be armed with the skills and knowledge to identify and manage it. Nurses have enormous potential to influence the course of, and patient's experience of, ACS. This is particularly important at a time when there is growing interest in the process and outcomes of nursing interventions, with a view to increasing the cost effectiveness and quality of care delivered.

The identification, treatment, and management of ACS is therefore likely to become an even more urgent issue in the future. If an early diagnosis is made, then recovery is the most common outcome. In most patients, the ACS is resolved completely within one to four weeks (American Psychiatric

Association, 1987). However, although it is by definition a transient phenomenon, it can also be a prelude to death and dementia in a small number of those affected. In any event, the length of hospital stay is likely to be increased, thus incurring additional cost to the health service.

Assessing a person who appears 'confused'

Assessing someone experiencing an ACS is a complex and skilled process. An individual's degree of disorientation, and the manifestations of this, are influenced by the time of day, environmental conditions, and physiological fluctuations. The person may interact differently away from his or her home environment and, unless relatives or close friends can give details, it can be difficult to establish clearly what significant changes have taken place in the individual's health and usual behaviour patterns. In addition, the person may be unable to give clear details and, in order to assess the situation fully, the nurse must use a full range of skills, particularly in building relationships, questioning techniques, and observation.

One difficulty in trying to assess someone experiencing ACS is that it is only that particular individual who understands the true reality of the experience. Assessment is therefore from an 'outsider looking in' perspective, which can distort the true reality as it is experienced. Descriptors used by nurses and doctors can also serve to distort further the reality (Foreman, 1991).

As Burnside (1988) states:

> The interview with a confused older person is perhaps one of the most difficult and draining of interactions with older clients. One has to realize that skill is acquired only by continually communicating with confused aged patients, trying to understand both the verbal and non-verbal messages, and developing a high level of patience and sensitivity (p. 201).

It is worth remembering that assessment conclusions can also be coloured by a nurse's expectations of how older people usually behave. For example, if a nurse expects a frail older person to sit quietly, someone who constantly walks and talks may be viewed as behaving unusually.

Key points in assessment

- Start assessing as soon as possible, and aim to assess the individual fully within 48 hours of admission.
- Question whether the individual is really disorientated, or whether

there are other factors that may be giving the appearance of confusion (such as hearing impairment, perceptual change, or language difficulty). Try to compensate for sensory impairment, and allow sufficient time for the individual to respond to questions.

- Try to establish what changes have taken place in the individual's health or behaviour, and when these change(s) began.
- Ascertain whether any specific change (such as acute illness, new drug treatment, or life event) triggered the change(s).
- Seek further information from those who may be able to give further details (such as family members, carers, GP, people or services who visit the individual at home, home matrons or warden).
- Assess for any indications of physical illness.
- Record significant biographical details that may help in the communication or assessment process.
- Try to establish how the individual usually functions, physically and cognitively.
- Assess the person's emotional state, how this changes, and what specifically triggers the change. Does the client have insight into situations? Are the responses relevant within reality as perceived by the patient? How long is the attention span? What are the patient's feelings about himself or herself?
- Listen to what the patient does not say as well as what he or she does.
- Record all baseline data to assist in ongoing assessment.
- Aim to identify persons at risk of developing ACS. These include people with known damage to the central nervous system, such as stroke, head trauma or tumour; those taking multiple medicines; those with cancer; and older people who have pre-existing cognitive or memory disturbance. ACS is common postoperatively. Labile or unusual behaviour may be the first sign (Sullivan and Fogel, 1986).
- Try to prevent the ACS developing, when possible.

Any comprehensive assessment will be ongoing and multifaceted. The elements within each assessment will be influenced by individual priorities, and the particular framework or model being used. As Wolanin and Phillips (1981) emphasize, an individual patient is always greater than the sum of the aspects within any assessment, no matter how systematic. However, for the purpose of analysis, the categories of assessment selected for discussion in this chapter are physiological, perceptual, cognitive, behavioural and biographical.

Physiological assessment

Clues to the cause of an ACS may be indicated by changes in;

- intake – of drugs (including prescribed medications or alcohol), fluids or foods
- output – of urine or faeces
- ability – to move around, function as previously, or maintain self-care

Baseline physiological measurements can also give clues, although it is important to appreciate that, particularly for people in their eighties and over, vital signs have different norms compared with those for younger people (Hogstel, 1994). For example, body temperature is not as sensitive an indicator as in younger people, and average temperatures may be lower in persons of advanced age. An elevated temperature may reflect an infection, especially in the chest or urinary tract, and a decreased temperature may reflect hypothermia, lack of body activity, or drugs that affect the thermoregulatory system, such as phenothiazines.

Pulse rate and respiration may be more sensitive indicators of infections, particularly if accompanied by other indicators such as general malaise.

For blood pressure to be a significant indicator, it is useful to know the person's usual level. With increased emphasis on health promotion in general practice, and with annual assessments of patients over seventy-five years of age, an obligation within the 1990 contract for GPs (Department of Health, 1989), the patient's GP will likely be a valuable source of health information. Blood pressure may be altered by drugs, especially antihypertensives, diuretics or tranquillizers.

The person's skin may give evidence of falls, infected areas and dryness, and also skin coldness, especially in the extremities and abdomen (hypothermia). However, because the skin in older people is often dry, it is not such a significant indicator of dehydration.

Indications of dehydration can be a dry mouth, the lack of a saliva pool under the tongue, and oliguria with urine of high specific gravity (especially as older people do not concentrate urine so easily). Other indicators may be a history of restricted access to fluids and increased haemoconcentration concurrent with hypovolaemia.

Changes in nutritional status may be evidenced by debility, loss of strength, or oedema. Weight loss, particularly if rapid, may be highlighted by loose skin, or loosely-fitting clothes. Problems with the teeth/dentures, gums or food manipulation may cause nutritional deficits, as can depressive illness, neurological and mobility deficits, or drugs/alcohol problems.

The urine should be tested, particularly for glucose, blood and protein. Abdominal and rectal examination should be carried out to establish whether the person is constipated.

Pain may also be an exacerbating factor, and nurses should carefully observe for evidence of this, bearing in mind that the experience of pain may be altered in older age (White, 1995).

Investigations may include a chest X-ray, or skull X-ray if the person has been falling. Blood tests may include full blood counts, blood cultures, thyroid function tests, urea and electrolytes. An electrocardiograph may be taken, and blood for cardiac enzymes. An electroencephalogram, and a computed tomographic scan can indicate focal or diffuse cerebral atrophy, intracranial masses, or hydrocephalus.

Assessment of perception

An older person's perceptions can be distorted by sight, hearing, tactile or olfactory impairment. This is particularly so following a cerebral vascular accident, when receptive dysphasia, expressive dysphasia and agnosia can affect perception and communication. Neurological changes following a stroke can also result in a person saying 'yes' when he or she means 'no', or moving to the right when trying to move the body to the left. Such changes should not be misinterpreted as mental confusion. The person's abilities should be maximized and alternative methods of communication should be sought for those with sight and hearing impairments.

Acute confusional state can result in a reduced ability to make sense of the environment and the current situation. It is also characterized by a reduced ability clearly to distinguish perceptions from imagery, dreams or hallucinations (Lipowski 1983). It can be helpful for nurses to try to understand the older person's current reality, although this may change and fluctuate, and to assess his or her perceptions within that reality.

Cognitive assessment

Cognitive processes, such as the ability to remember, reason, problem-solve, and sustain goal-directed behaviour for any length of time, are characteristically affected by ACS. Thinking may become disorganized and fragmented (Lipowski, 1983), and the patient's conversation may become tangential or scattered, giving the impression that he or she is distracted (Zimberg and Berenson, 1990).

The person's ability to organize thought content, the ability to think abstractly, and knowledge of current events, may provide helpful information on current cognitive functioning (Inaba-Roland and Maricle, 1992).

One of the problems in assessing cognition is that, in order for the patient to respond appropriately and effectively, the requested information must be of relevance. The older person must see the point in the questions being asked, be interested in what is being said, and maintain this interest long enough to retrieve the information being asked. This is particularly important with patients who are emotional, anxious, withdrawn, depressed or suspicious. They may suspect that the nurse is trying to make a fool of them (Wolanin and Phillips 1981). People who are ill also have preoccupations, such as physical symptoms or concerns about their health, which are paramount in their minds, and thus distract them from conversation.

Attention and attention span are usually affected. People experiencing ACS may be either inattentive or hypervigilant. In both states, the person is unable to focus on what is occurring and may lose concentration, interrupt or wander mentally (Zimberg and Berenson, 1990).

All aspects of memory can be impaired by ACS. Recent memory is characteristically more impaired than remote memory. Recent recall may be impaired as a result of a reduced attention span, with the result that, because a person cannot recall an event or interaction, he or she may deny that it ever occurred (Zimberg and Berenson, 1990). The ability to learn is reduced (Lipowski, 1983). Recognition is a cruder form of memory than recall. When assessing memory, it may be helpful to offer a range of answers for the patient. Although he or she may not be able to recall with only the question as stimulus, he or she may be able to select the correct response from the alternatives. It can be useful to test recent memory, remote memory, recall and recognition, and to note whether the patient admits being unable to recall, or confabulates (Wolanin and Phillips, 1981).

Judgement can be assessed by observing whether the person uses objects in the environment appropriately.

The ability to follow simple commands can also be assessed in day-to-day care.

Although orientation is not a cognitive function as such, it is an outcome of healthy cognitive functioning. Global orientation, to time, place and person, is not usually impaired until the ACS is severe, but immediate orientation to the surrounding environment and time of day will usually be affected (Zimberg and Berenson, 1990).

When assessing a patient's orientation to time it is useful to remember that there can be different perceptions of time. As well as the date/hour reality, there may also be time perception in an individual's own internal body rhythms, and also in personal events or times. All three of these may be different. Time may also be perceived differently within a different environment, such as hospital. Another interesting aspect concerns those patients who are from different cultures, because language may express time differently (for example, some Asian cultures perceive past and present as continuous).

Orientation to place may be more accurately assessed by asking a patient for impressions of the present place, and how it differs from his or her home.

Orientation to person may present problems because the term 'person' can encompass not only time but also the many roles a person assumes throughout life. It may be more helpful for the nurse to ask the patient who he or she is, what he or she is, and what he or she does (Wolanin and Phillips, 1981).

Foreman (1991) reminds us that, as typical hospital environments have a marked effect on the 'diurnal biological rhythms of daily human life', even patients who are not acutely confused often experience some disorientation while they are hospitalized (Foreman, 1991, p. 13). Physiological factors such as pain, fatigue or sleep deprivation, can also affect mental state.

Behavioural assessment

A person experiencing ACS may be predominantly hyperactive or hypoactive, or may switch from one of these extremes to the other in the course of a day. Both nonverbal behaviour and speech are affected (Lipowski, 1983).

When trying to understand an older person's behaviour, it is extremely helpful to have insight into how he or she has previously responded in similar circumstances. It can also be helpful to try to place behaviour within the context of the person's current reality. When viewed within the individual's current reality, the behaviour is often logical.

Some behaviours, particularly agitated motor behaviours, may be a manifestation of the cause of the ACS (such as cerebral hypoxia). Foreman (1991) suggests that a person's concentration and attention span may be a more useful indicator of mental processes than orientation or psychomotor behaviour.

Biographical assessment

Biographical details may offer significant clues to behaviour or speech content in ACS. Such details include cultural background, religious beliefs, work experiences, significant family members or friends, reactions to life changes (such as retirement), past coping strategies, and recent losses. These may be important, not for the events themselves, but for the significance of the experience to the individual older person (Schofield, 1994).

Assessment tools

Bowling (1991, 1995) describes many instruments that may be used to assess mental orientation. They can be helpful in assessing changes in, for example, mental functioning. These can aid the objectivity of an assessment and many can be used in quick and fairly reliable assessments of whether an older person has significant cognitive impairment. They should be used with caution, however, as they do not in themselves provide a full cognitive assessment or allow a diagnosis to be made. In fact, it is dangerous to assume that they do diagnose. Various psychological tests, particularly those concerning memory, can be used, but these are fraught with methodological difficulties.

The Mini-Mental State Examination (MMSE) (Folstein et al., 1975) is one of the most widely used instruments for screening for cognitive impairment. It covers orientation, registration, attention and calculation, recall and language. Each item is scored; a total score of less than thirty indicates cognitive impairment. The reading and writing elements of the test may present difficulty for people with visual impairment (Bowling, 1995). The MMSE has been demonstrated to be valid and reliable (Foreman, 1991, 1993).

The ability to carry out practical tests can also be assessed by activity of living scales and overall behaviours can be assessed on scales such as the Crichton Royal Behavioural Rating Scale and the Clifton Assessment Procedures for the Elderly (CAPE). Foreman's (1991) study used the MMSE alongside behavioural scales, and suggested a close relationship between the cognitive and behavioural changes when ACS is observed by nurses. Foreman's results also suggested that two types of instruments may be needed in nursing practice and research, one to detect the onset of confusion (i.e. a screening tool with cognitive and perceptual dimensions) and another to determine the level of confusion (i.e. a tool with more behavioural dimensions of confusion) (Vermeersch, 1991).

Management of acute confusional state

Management of the ACS is very much a joint effort between nursing and medical staff. Either group may have been instrumental in making a preliminary diagnosis, although generally the quest for the underlying cause is the remit of the medical staff. Nevertheless, nurses will be involved in collecting samples for diagnostic tests and carrying out prescribed medical care, alongside their own responsibilities for managing the cognitive and behavioural disturbances characteristic of the condition.

While full recovery of the patient is obviously the prime desirable outcome, the person's safety, and that of staff and other patients, is considered to be the essential feature of effective care. In addition, the maintenance of dignity, self-esteem and self-confidence, in situations that can all too readily lead to ridicule and shame, are also important aspects of the management process. Manipulation of the environment, attention to communication and ensuring continuity are considered to be the key areas for focusing nursing care (Sugden and Saxby, 1985). Manipulation of the physical environment can contribute to the prevention of physical injury of the patient, or to other patients and staff. The patient is at risk because of severe disorientation and disorganized behaviour. In addition to the usual safety measures, other strategies are worth considering. The patient's bed should be placed at its lowest level and the use of bed-rails confined to those who are insufficiently agile to climb over them or through the gap towards the foot of the bed. Another option might be to place the mattress on the floor, although there are benefits and disadvantages of taking such actions. Although this would prevent the patient from falling out of bed, it contradicts ideas surrounding normality and continuity (most people do not sleep on the floor) and, as a result, might well increase the patient's disorientation. Furthermore, attending to a patient at floor level is hardly conducive to safe manual handling.

Disorientation to time, place and person usually occurs in that order. It tends to be worse at night, when the reduction in the level of stimuli, often exacerbated by age-related sensory deficits in sight and hearing, fail to provide sufficient orientation cues. A single room with a night light, set at a level that does not produce sharp contrasts and shadows, may provide an environment in which distractions are kept to a minimum, enabling the patient to settle (Williams et al., 1979). Alternatively, the patient may appear more calm and in control when sitting in a comfortable armchair in a well-lit day room.

Disturbance of the sleep–wake cycle, with insomnia and daytime sleepiness (known as sundowning in the American literature), is one of the diagnostic criteria of ACS cited by the American Psychiatric Society. Wolanin and Phillips (1981) suggest that causes may be found by studying events at the end of the patient's day. They cite fatigue, incontinence, increased noise, decreased light, pain and fewer staff on duty. These are mostly conditions that are amenable to nursing intervention and are therefore preventable.

The use of colour to distinguish different parts of the ward (for example, for walls or furnishings), and encouraging the patient to bring in personal and familiar belongings, can provide points of reference that help to orientate the patient to his or her bed area. Lavatory doors can be colour-coded or labelled with large lettering for easy recognition. Patients can be shown the location of their own personal commode or urinal, and this information can be repeated at intervals. Williams et al. (1979, 1985), in a study of postoperative orthopaedic patients, found that disruptions in patient's elimination routines contributed to ACS. In addition, for patients in the same studies, the availability of timepieces, calendars and access to TV and newspapers, were instrumental in reducing the level of confusion.

Attention to communication in the form of reality orientation has been given credence by the work of Folsom (1968) and Holden and Woods (1982), although these were studies of people with irreversible mental impairment. The work of Williams et al. (1985) appears to be one of the few that demonstrates the effectiveness of orientation techniques (although they do not use the term 'reality orientation') in the care of patients with ACS. McMahon (1988), however, argues against the use of reality orientation as a special therapeutic approach, making the point that effective communication techniques are integral to effective nursing care and, as such, would be structured to account for the patient's level of functioning.

Foreman (1993) suggests that a reduced ability to maintain attention to external stimuli is the primary deficit of ACS. Altered attention and concentration may be evidenced by: distracted and disjointed conversations; an inability to focus on tasks and self-care; restless, agitated motor behaviour, such as picking at the bedclothes; and seeming constantly on guard, alert and fearful. Interactions from staff should be directed towards one thing at a time, focusing on that which has immediate relevance to the situation. This could involve reinforcing information on nurses' intentions and purpose of care, medications being offered and the need for intravenous infusions. Any information should be provided in clear, concise chunks, using simple terms and adopting a calm voice tone while being face to face with the patient.

Assistance with essential self-care activities will also be required until the ACS begins to resolve. Nurses should concentrate their efforts on priorities such as drinking and eating and assisting with elimination, in order to maintain continence. The person with ACS is unlikely to tolerate lengthy hygiene procedures, although attention to correct dress and the prevention of immodesty is integral to the maintenance of dignity. When approaching the patient, care should be taken not to startle him or her. A voice tone that expresses concern and simple, honest communication, is more likely to have a calming influence and reduce the patient's fear.

Short-term memory loss may also be in evidence. The patient may be unable to recall recent information, such as the reason for the admission to hospital, and may also be unable to remember recent meaningful events, such as being admitted to hospital, visits by friends and family, or the location of personal items. Each time contact is made with the patient, it is necessary to reinforce that he or she is in hospital and for how long, the reason for admission, the time of day, and who you are. Of course, this needs to be done simply and with pauses, in order not to overload the patient with information. It is important to avoid complex instructions and requests to make decisions, as the patient may have difficulty in responding.

Apprehension, fear and loss of control, suspiciousness and paranoia can occur as a result of altered thought processes. Often as a result of careful active listening, fears and anxieties can be identified in what seems to be, on the face of it, irrelevant and incoherent speech. Care involves assessing the patient's feelings towards staff and the need to be in hospital. Distortions in thoughts and feelings need to be clarified and the nature and purpose of each nursing intervention explained. The patient should be reassured that the staff are concerned about his or her welfare and will not cause any harm. Misunderstandings and misinterpretations of events can lead to expressions of anger and hostility, or threats towards staff, culminating in physical assault, if the behaviour is not well managed in the early stages. Anger should be acknowledged verbally, followed by reassurance that the nurse is concerned about the patient's feelings and needs. The nurse could ask what help is needed, followed by the reinforcement of a desire to be helpful. A further option is to suggest that the patient has a desire to receive help and not cause any violence: 'You want us to help you. You really don't want to hurt someone' (Zimberg and Berenson, 1990).

Perceptual disturbances in the form of illusions and hallucinations are also characteristic of ACS. The former tends to be more common than the latter. Illusions have a basis in reality. For example, a woman pointed to a blue woollen blanket lying folded on her bed, saying that it was the jumper she was knitting for her son. It was easy enough to show her the blanket, saying, 'Yes, it looks like a jumper, but see, it's your bed blanket.' Sometimes illusions can be quite frightening. For example, a male patient in an orthopaedic ward described seeing funerals and mourners. His bed was near the entrance to the ward and it is very likely that he was witnessing the arrival and departure of trolleys transporting patients to and from theatre and from the accident and emergency department (Schofield, 1993). Hallucinations have no basis in reality and can vary from being pleasant, such as descriptions of visits from dead relatives, or frightening and disturbing experiences.

Management of the patient with ACS is often accompanied by many ethical dilemmas for nurses, particularly when the person becomes disruptive and violent to other patients and staff. When patients are able to understand, make and express a choice, then, in the majority of circumstances, nurses must support this choice (British Medical Association and Royal College of Nursing, 1995). However, in circumstances where patients are cognitively impaired (albeit temporarily), they cannot be considered responsible for their own actions. In such cases, the law decrees that the medical consultant in charge of their care must act in the patients' best interests and 'do what is reasonable in all the circumstances to care for that person and to safeguard and promote his or her welfare' (English Law Commission, 1993). Such actions are often devolved to nursing staff, although with little explicit guidance about what is the best course of action.

Furthermore, if the safety and comfort of other patients and staff are threatened, nurses may feel that they must take a utilitarian approach, thus acting for the good of the majority but restricting the freedom of the affected patient. Nurses may then feel the need to resort to some form of restraint. This may simply be leaving the patient in a low chair, from which he or she is unable to rise without assistance, then, through a range of other tactics, eventually resorting to the use of chemical restraint.

The Royal College of Nursing's group, Focus on Older People, Nursing and Mental Health (1992) and Counsel and Care (1992), recognize that nurses are sometimes left with little or no option but to use restraint, but that it should be used as a last resort after all the patient-centred therapeutic approaches already discussed have been exhausted. It would also need to be carried out with the full cooperation of medical colleagues. To this end, Focus on Older People (1992) and Counsel and Care (1993) have produced guidelines on the use of restraint, which emphasize the importance of documenting actions and rationales and limiting the duration of the restraint period.

Ensuring continuity and minimizing disruption to the patient's normal life patterns is the third key area for therapeutic input. Continuity of care is best provided by as few carers as possible; primary and team nursing are therefore suited to this. Encouraging visits, and even overnight stays from family and friends, is another important way of keeping in touch with home and normality. However, in the first instance, visitors are often distressed to see their loved one so obviously disturbed. It is important to look out for people when they come to visit, so that they can be prepared for such changes. The nurse should ensure that they are aware that the ACS is caused by physical illness, and that it is of a temporary nature.

Visitors will need to know if and how the condition has affected the patient's thought processes and behaviour, and how best to communicate. Nursing staff should be present to give guidance and support until visitors feel able to cope on their own. If it is not possible to visit, contact can be maintained by telephone. Hearing a familiar voice may contribute to reducing the confused person's anxiety and stress. Photographs of family members and pets also provide reference points. Furthermore, knowledge of the patient's past and present life gleaned from family and friends can provide topics for simple conversation, initiated by the nurse. The sense of self can be reinforced by patients wearing their own clothing and being able to view themselves in a mirror.

Finally, on resolution of the ACS, the patient may be left with feelings of unresolved fear and anxiety, a loss of dignity, and apprehension at their temporary loss of control. It is important that the nurse should ensure that the patient understands that the ACS was caused by a physical illness that has now been treated, and that the episode was of a temporary nature. The nurse should also offer to facilitate the patient's exploration of the experience if desired. A small exploratory study into patients' retrospective experience of ACS has demonstrated their willingness to talk about it (Schofield, 1993).

Conclusion

Acute confusional state is a complex phenomenon, with a variety of definitions that emphasize different behavioural and cognitive manifestations. It is a common symptom of illness in older people and is often the only indication that something is wrong. It is the most common psychiatric syndrome found in general hospital wards, and significant numbers of older people are likely to experience acute confusion at some time during hospitalization. It presents as a medical emergency, and treatment consists of removal of the underlying cause.

In addition to the stress of physical illness and the experience of hospitalization, the alterations in cognitive, emotional and behavioural functioning that accompany ACS may cause the older person to lose a sense of control and self-esteem, and cause emotional stress to the family, friends and carers. Nurses have a vital role in prevention, recognition, assessment and treatment, but also in providing physical, psychological and environment support. Once the ACS has resolved, nurses can assist patients to reflect on the experience, and to place events and actions into an appropriate context. This can help to resolve the bewilderment, embarrassment and perceived loss of control that many older people experience.

To date, the majority of research into ACS has concentrated on professional perspectives. There is a need for further work, focusing on the older person's subjective meaning of the experience of ACS, thus developing a more comprehensive understanding of this important health and quality of life issue for older people.

References

American Psychiatric Association. (1987). *Diagnostic and Statistical Manual of Mental Disorders*, 3rd ed. rev. pp. 100–103, Washington, DC: APA.

Bowling, A. (1991). *Measuring Health: a Review of Quality of Life Measurement Scales*. Milton Keynes: Open University Press.

Bowling, A. (1995). *Measuring Disease: a Review of Disease-specific Quality of Life Measurement Scales*. Milton Keynes: Open University Press.

British Medical Association and Royal College of Nursing. (1995). *The Older Person: Consent and Care*. London: British Medical Association.

Brooking, J. (1986). Depression and other mental disorders in the elderly. In *Nursing Elderly People*. (S. Redfern, ed.), pp. 241–254. Edinburgh: Churchill Livingstone.

Burnside, I. (1988). *Nursing the Aged: a Self-care Approach*, 3rd ed., New York: McGraw Hill.

Counsel and Care. (1992). *What if They Hurt Themselves: a Discussion Document on the Uses and Abuses of Restraint in Residential Care and Nursing Homes for Older People*, London: Counsel and Care.

Counsel and Care. (1993). *The Right to Take Risks: Model Policies, Guidance to Staff and Training Material on Restraint and Risk-taking in Residential Care and Nursing Homes for Older People*. London: Counsel and Care.

Department of Health. (1989). *Terms of Service for Doctors in General Practice*. London: HMSO.

English Law Commission. (1993). *Mentally Incapacitated Adults and Decision-Making: a New Jurisdiction*. London: English Law Commission.

Focus on Older People, Nursing and Mental Health. (1992). *Focus on Restraint: Guidelines on the Use of Restraint in the Care of Older People*, 2nd ed., London: Royal College of Nursing.

Folsom, J. C. (1968). Reality orientation for the elderly mental patient. *J. Geriatr. Psychiatry*, 1, 291–307.

Folstein, M. F., Folstein, S. E. and McHugh P. R. (1975). 'Mini-mental state': a practical guide for grading the cognitive state of patients for clinicians. *J. Psychiatr. Res.*, 12, 189–198.

Foreman, M. D. (1991). The cognitive and behavioural nature of acute confusional states. *Scholarly Inquiry Nurs. Pract.*, 5, 3–16.

Foreman, M. (1993). Acute confusion in the elderly. *Annu. Rev. Nurs. Res.*, **11**, 3–30.

Hogstel, M. O. (1994). Vital signs are really vital in the old-old. *Geriatr. Nurs.*, **15**, 252–255.

Holden, U. P. and Woods, R. T. (1982). *Reality Orientation: Psychological Approaches to the Confused Elderly.* London: Churchill Livingstone.

Inaba-Roland, K. E. and Maricle, R. A. (1992). Assessing delirium in the acute care setting. *Heart Lung*, **21**, 48–55.

Lipowski, Z. J. (1983). Transient cognitive disorders (delirium, acute confusional states) in the elderly. *Am. J. Psychiatry*, **140**, 1427–1435.

Lucas, M. J. and Folstein, M. F. (1980). Nursing assessment of mental disorders on a general medical unit. *J. Psychiatr. Nurs. Ment. Health Serv.*, **18**, 31–33.

McMahon, R. (1988). The 24-hour reality orientation type of approach to the confused elderly: a minimum standard for care. *J. Adv. Nurs.*, **13**, 693–700.

Palmateer, L. M. and McCartney, J. R. (1985). Do nurses know when patients have cognitive deficits? *J. Gerontol. Nurs.*, **11**, 6–16.

Raisin, J. H. (1990). Confusion. *Nurs. Clin. North Am.*, **25**, 909–918.

Schofield, I. (1993). *A Small Exploratory Study of the Reaction of Older People to an Episode of Delirium.* [dissertation]. London: King's College.

Schofield, I. (1994). Using a historical approach to care. *Elderly Care*, **6**(6), 14–15.

Sugden, J. and Saxby, P. J. (1985). The confused elderly patient. *Nursing*, **35**, 1022–1024.

Sullivan N. and Fogel, B. S. (1986). Could this be delirium? *Am. J. Nurs.*, **83**, 1359–1363.

Vermeersch, P. E. H. (1991). Response to 'The cognitive and behavioural nature of acute confusional states'. *Scholarly Inquiry Nurs. Pract.*, **5**, 17–20.

White I. (1995). Pain control. In *Foundations in Nursing Theory and Practice.* (H. B. M. Heath, ed.) p. 546. London: Mosby.

Williams, M. A., Holloway, J. R., Winn, M. C. et al. (1979). Nursing activities and acute confusional states in elderly hip-fractured patients. *Nurs. Res.*, **28**, 25–35.

Williams, M. A. Campbell, E. B., Raynor, W. J. et al. (1985). Reducing acute confusional states in elderly patients with hip fractures. *Res. Nurs. Health*, **8**, 329–337

Wolanin, M. O. (1973). *Confusion in the Elderly.* (Paper presented at the Gerontological Research Conference.) New York: Blue Mountain Lake.

Wolanin, M. O. and Phillips, L. R. (1981). *Confusion, Prevention and Care*, St Louis, MO: Mosby.

Zimberg, M. and Berenson, S. (1990). Delirium in patients with cancer: nursing assessment and intervention. *Oncol. Nurs. Forum*, **17**, 529–538.

7

Depression in old age

Nigel Harrison

Introduction

This chapter considers depression in older people. It contrasts differing definitions, methods of classification and types of depression. The causes and frequency of depression are considered and possible methods for assessment. The main body of the chapter focuses on a nursing framework for helping these individuals, and a selection of physical, psychological and social therapies that can be used.

The aim of the chapter is to give the reader the opportunity to examine the concept of depression in older people and the therapeutic role of the nurse.

Background

A common belief is that depression is a natural result of ageing. Murphy et al. (1986) assert that most elderly people are not depressed, although younger people might hold stereotypical views of older people being miserable and sad. Depression in old age is a possible source of stigma and has become linked to older people as unwanted, unpleasant and unenviable.

Defining depression

Depression has been defined in the *Mosby Medical, Nursing and Allied Health Dictionary* (1994) as 'an abnormal emotional state characterized by exaggerated feelings of sadness, melancholy, dejection, worthlessness, emptiness and hopelessness, which are inappropriate and out of proportion to reality'. In contrast, Rowe (1983) describes depression as 'a social construct, a prison where the individual is both the suffering prisoner and the cruel jailer, iso-lated, filled with fear, anger, guilt and despair'.

Frequency of depression

On average, between ten and twenty per cent of those aged over sixty-five years have a clinical syndrome of depression (Gearing et al., 1988). Most peo-ple with affective illnesses, who are over seventy, will be experiencing a re-currence of depression which commenced earlier in their life (Post, 1981). However, as the numbers of older people increase, it is to be expected that the incidence of depression will also rise. Gearing et al. (1988) state that offi-cial services are aware only of a small percentage of the total number of older people with mental health problems. This emphasizes the importance of careful screening in order to ensure that vulnerable older people are identi-fied and appropriate intervention is made available prior to their situations becoming worse.

Classification of depression

There have been several attempts to classify depression or 'affective disorder' using medical and scientific approaches. Beaumont and Anfield (1983) con-sider that current classifications are not helpful as they 'package people into specific categories for the sake of diagnostic purposes'. An alternative model is to take an ethnographic approach, which emphasizes life experiences and considers individual needs.

Classification according to cause

Classification of depression according to the cause includes 'exogenous' (pri-mary) and endogenous (secondary) types. In endogenous depression, the cause is believed to be unknown, although influenced by genetic or bio-chemical factors. Conversely, exogenous, or reactive depression, is consid-ered to be milder and caused by external stress such as bereavement, stress and reduced social support, although stressful life events can also precede endogenous depression (Blazer, 1993). Wilkinson (1989) describes 'primary depression' as having no obvious precipitating mental or physical factors, whereas 'secondary depression' originates from physical or psychotic illness such as drug or alcohol abuse.

Norman (1991) states that age-related changes assume increasing impor-tance in influencing an individual's internal and external environment.

These changes include the development of physical disease, genetic influences and social stressors involving bereavement, loneliness and lack of social support.

Further views on the causes of depression suggest a 'cognitive learning theory' approach, in which it is believed that negative thoughts, errors in thinking and depressive patterns of thinking exist (Holmes and Rahe, 1967; Beck, 1976; Kendell, 1976; Murphy, 1982). In addition, Seligman (1975) states that 'learned helplessness' can occur as a result of inescapable stress.

Classification according to symptoms

The classification of depression according to symptoms is usually described as psychotic or neurotic. Psychotic depression, including manic depressive psychosis, can be severe and include delusions, hallucinations, disordered thought, socially unacceptable behaviour and a lack of insight. Neurotic depression is less severe and follows a distressing experience and preoccupation (for example, the loss of a pet or of possessions following a burglary). Agitation and related illnesses may accompany neurotic depression such as hypochondriasis or agoraphobia (Wilkinson, 1989). Post (1981) suggests that many older people with neurotic depression see their doctor for physical complaints, and are often only seen by psychiatrists when treatment has been unsuccessful or following attempted suicide (parasuicide).

Classification following the course of an illness

Depression is one of the most frequent psychiatric syndromes among physically ill older people (Blazer, 1993). It is often unrecognized and accounts for increased morbidity and mortality rates. Bipolar depression refers to severe episodes of the illness, in which there are alternating episodes of depression and mania. Williams (1992) states that bipolar depression is far less common, occurring in one in ten depressive illnesses. In unipolar depression, the mood alternates between low mood and normal, and does not include manic episodes. When there are physical problems (for example, visual or hearing impairment, and complex histories with multiple pathologies), depression may be masked and underlie unexplained physical disorders such as chronic pain. Low mood and other symptoms characteristic of depression are not always clear (Wilkinson, 1989).

A consistency between the classifications is the distinction made between two opposite poles. Professionals tend to indicate whether the depression is mild, moderate or severe without considering the relevance of a client's own experience.

Assessment

Blazer (1993) believes that many elderly individuals who experience depressive symptoms do not contact mental health or any other professionals. If they are seen by health care workers, depressive symptoms are often overlooked. Older people often present with a complex range of physical and mental symptoms and problems. It can often be difficult to distinguish between their various emotions, such as anger, anxiety and depression. Similarly, Post (1981) asserts that older people who are suffering from neurotic depression rarely seek help or advice from health professionals.

The nurse is in a key position to assist in the assessment of these older people and to determine the primary and secondary features of depression. The Royal College of Nursing (1990) provides guidelines for the assessment of older people, which serve as a useful foundation to help to identify specific areas requiring more in-depth assessment.

Rawlins and Heacock (1993) advise mental health nurses to structure assessments using a holistic approach, which acknowledges the different dimensions of an integrated and functioning person. This involves the nurse assessing clients' psychological, physical, social, environmental and spiritual needs.

Cognitive behavioural assessment

There are a number of cognitive behavioural assessment rating scales for depression, such as the Hamilton Rating Scale for Depression, the Cognitive Style Inventory, the Dysfunctional Attitude Scale and the Hopelessness Scale (Williams, 1992). Perhaps the most well known is the Beck Depression Inventory (Beck et al., 1961). This consists of a series of twenty-one statements for assessing existing levels of depression. Those with depression characteristically score higher than nondepressed people. An individual completes the inventory by selecting one of five possible choices in relation to the way in which they feel or think. Murphy et al. (1984) have used this as a way of defining the level of depression from 'not depressed' to 'severely depressed'. When used as an initial baseline assessment and at regular intervals, it enables treatment or intervention to be monitored and changed as required.

Nonverbal behaviour

Ellgring (1989) considers that nonverbal behaviour in mental illness is relevant because it plays a central role in the mutual understanding and communication between the patient and others. Nonverbal behaviour can be used for diagnostic purposes and for measuring the effectiveness of therapies. However, pressure to validate such observations empirically, and to be able to quantify an assessment, has led to efforts in the USA to develop rating scales for measuring nonverbal behaviour in depression. Ellgring (1989) warns that nonverbal behaviour can change daily. Generalizations about a person's mental state should not therefore be drawn solely from these observations. In addition, it is important to be sensitive to differences in the age, gender and culture of the older person. It is generally accepted that verbal characteristics and statements are less subtle and therefore easier to rate.

Blazer (1993) stresses that observable signs may be especially relevant in older people, who may not volunteer their symptoms or may be so depressed that they are unable to respond during an interview.

Pitt (1988) outlines the features of depression, clarifying that, to make a diagnosis of depression, four or more of these need to be present nearly every day for two weeks:

- Prominent and persistent mood disturbance
- Loss of interest and pleasure in usual activities and pastimes
- Poor appetite and weight loss; may include constipation (increased appetite and weight gain is not common in older people)
- Insomnia: includes difficulty in getting to sleep or early morning wakening, and sometimes waking in the middle of the night, with difficulty in returning to sleep
- Psychomotor agitation or retardation: includes restlessness, pacing, hand wringing, fidgeting, moaning and groaning, or sluggish and slow speech and movements
- Decreased sexual drive
- Energy loss, fatigue and social withdrawal
- Feelings of worthlessness, guilt and low self-esteem (nihilistic and hypochondriacal delusions and auditory hallucinations may exist in psychotic depression)
- Inability to concentrate, slowed thinking, forgetfulness and indecisiveness
- Recurrent thoughts of death and suicide

Physical interventions

Medication

Pleuvry and Snowdon (1988) provide an overview of the main types of drugs prescribed for treating depression, these include tricyclic antidepressants, monoamine oxidase inhibitors (MAOIs) and 5-HT reuptake inhibitors.

There are a number of tricyclic antidepressants that are suitable for older people. These are most commonly used because of low toxicity and side effects. Most take between two and four weeks to reach therapeutic blood levels.

With MAOIs, the nurse has a responsibility to educate the patient and re-inforce the need for a selective dietary intake. Examples include the avoidance of cheese, pickled herrings, broad bean pods, banana, ice cream and meat extracts, including beef spreads. There is also the possibility of adverse drug interactions, requiring the avoidance of certain medications. MAOI treatment cards are issued to reinforce health advice so that a hypertensive crisis can be avoided. The main side effect is postural hypotension, so the nurse needs to teach the patient to stand up slowly (Pleuvry and Snowdon, 1988).

In 1987, Prozac, a 5-HT reuptake inhibitor arrived on the market and was heralded as the new 'designer drug' for treating depression, bulimia nervosa and obsessive compulsive disorder. Pharmaceutical manufacturers claim that there are only minor side effects and no physical addictive properties, and that there is safety in overdose (Healy, 1993). This may be attractive to some older people who want an immediate improvement of their symptoms when they think that they only have a limited life expectancy.

Anxiolytics and night sedation may also be given to control anxiety and sleep disturbance, although the increasing incidence and recent publicity of addiction has caused these drugs to be used more cautiously. Lithium carbonate and neuroleptics may also to be administered to control mania and psychoses (Pleuvry and Snowdon, 1988). Healy (1993) offers further information on specific drugs currently used in the treatment of depression and mania.

Electroconvulsive therapy

Electroconvulsive therapy (ECT), although used less frequently today, is an alternative therapy for severely depressed older people. Indications for its use include (Benbow, 1991; Blazer, 1993):

- Risk of suicide
- Sleep disturbance
- Refusal to eat resulting in weight loss
- Psychotic symptoms
- Lack of response to antidepressants and/or psychotherapy
- Manic symptoms
- Previous positive responsiveness to ECT

The preparation of an older person for ECT needs to include diagnostic tests to eradicate possible complications (i.e. baseline mental state examination, history of previous treatment for depression, chest radiography, electrocardiography, full blood count, CT scan and/or multiresonance imaging). Blazer (1993) also outlines the contraindications to be considered, before proceeding with ECT. These include:

- The degree of frailty of the older person
- Whether there are any lesions within the central nervous system (thereby augmenting the risk of increased intracranial pressure)
- Cardiovascular disease and unsuitability for anaesthesia due to respiratory disease
- Possible complications due to existing medication

In addition, the nurse needs to assist and support these patients, providing explanations and reassurance with regard to the technique of ECT and what to expect afterwards. A nurse needs to be knowledgeable and able to respond in a language that is understandable to each individual. It is good practice for the named nurse to provide time for the patient to ask questions.

Exercise

Dzyak (1990) believes that physical exercise for older people has gained acceptance by health care professionals, but scientific evidence for its use is sparse. One example includes a high-stepping exercise programme, which can promote strength and self-esteem in older people (Case-McAleer, 1993). Weinstein (1986) discusses the benefits of swimming and water activities in older people, and Beck et al. (1992) advocates the use of exercise as a method of intervention for managing aggression and behavioural problems. Nurses are able to use exercise for health promotion and disease prevention purposes because they have the technical skills, the frequency of contact and credibility with older adults. Correct assessment and adherence to protocols are, however, essential (Topp, 1991).

Psychological interventions

Psychological therapies offer personal growth and insight, and teach coping strategies for managing depressive episodes. Blazer (1993) advocates the use of different types of psychotherapy for treating depression in later life. Nurses may initiate any of these interventions as autonomous professionals or work alongside other health care workers in this field. Many community psychiatric nurses have undertaken training in counselling and family therapy. Nurses are now in a position to establish themselves as independent nurse practitioners, offering specific skills for managing depression in older people. Referrals may come from other nurses' and health care professionals on a sessional basis as part of these nurses' extended role (Sheehan, 1994).

Cognitive behavioural therapies

Gilbert (1992) outlines how a cognitive interpersonal approach to counselling can be used for treating depression. One method is to explore the opportunities for an alternative life style. The older person is asked to examine a recent event, through the use of open, probing and hypothetical questions. This then helps them to understand the links between their thoughts, beliefs and emotions, and how these relate to being depressed. Gilbert (1992) stresses the importance of creating a situation in which the exploration is a collaborative and friendly experience and not an interrogation. He points out that timing is crucial, so that, if a patient wishes to vent painful feelings, then highly focused work such as the use of the triple column technique, may need to be held back so that it does not hinder any therapeutic intervention. Complex chains can be triggered by such exercises and it is useful to deal with one theme at a time when a person needs assistance to deal with shame, guilt, ideals or envy (Dryden, 1989; Gilbert, 1992).

In order to achieve this, it is important to look for key words used by patients. This can indicate their thoughts about themselves and their underlying beliefs. Nurses are in an ideal position to probe sensitively and explore these beliefs, emotions and behaviour. A person may admit to feeling unworthy of love and companionship from others and ashamed of the pain and suffering that his or her depression is causing to close family members. A long-term aim would to be to challenge some of these beliefs that the person has identified and enable him or her to think and/or behave differently.

Williams (1992) and Beck et al. (1979) outline a number of other interventions and cognitive behavioural techniques that a nurse can use:

- *Graded task assignment:* Specific behaviours are organized in a graduated series of goals to be achieved with increasing complexity.
- *Cognitive reorganization:* This involves pinpointing cognitive distortions and demonstrating their invalidity.
- *Scheduling activities:* This involves organizing and encouraging participation in a number of structured activities throughout the day to relieve unpleasant feelings.

- *Mastery and pleasure:* This requires the patient to keep a diary of events that have been successful or given pleasure, to demonstrate progress and achievement.
- *Cognitive rehearsal:* Here, the barriers that prevent the patient from achieving a goal are discussed, using a hypothetical situation.
- *Alternative therapy:* Here the client is encouraged to consider alternative explanations of their experiences, which challenges negative thinking and offers a more accurate viewpoint.
- *Homework tasks:* Specific realistic activities are set at the end of a session, for achievement by the next meeting. This includes logging the thoughts and feelings attached to an experience and the rationale response for comparison and later discussion.

Counselling

One definition states that the task of counselling is to give the patient an opportunity to explore, discover and clarify ways of living more satisfyingly and resourcefully (British Association for Counselling, 1984). The British Association for Counselling Code of Ethics (1989) makes a clear distinction between counselling and the use of counselling skills. Counselling is said to be characterized by the existence of an explicit and formal contract between the counsellor and the patient, where there is no conflict of roles. In contrast, counselling skills are said to enhance communication skills with someone, but without taking on the role of a counsellor. Nurses can use specific counselling skills, such as listening, attending, questioning, reflection, paraphrasing and summarizing, to encourage patients to explore their feelings in relation to recent problems. Some nurses need to accept the limitations of their role and refer patients on. However, Scrutton (1989) states that the professionalization of counselling denies that the techniques involved are a set of skills that are essentially a simple and very human means of helping people in trouble. He views a counsellor of older people as a carer and friend, involving close relationships, empathy and good communication.

There are different models of counselling, which outline the processes involved in counselling and offer frameworks for the nurse and other helpers to follow. Egan (1994) suggests a three-stage model of helping. This involves a process of exploring and defining the problem, understanding and setting goals, then following through a plan of action. Nelson-Jones (1993) advocates using a five-stage model, which aims to empower patients in developing life skills. Most models use a problem-solving approach and involve similar progressive stages.

Table 7.1 Comparison of two counselling models

Egan (1994)	Nelson-Jones (1993)
Explore and define problems	Develop the relationship; identify and clarify problems
	Assess problems and redefine them as skills to be achieved by the patient
Understand and set goals	State working goals and plan interventions
Action taken to implement goals set	Action by the patient
	End and consolidate with self-helping skills

Jacobs (1988) suggests information that may be sought when assessing a person's suitability for counselling. This is relevant for assessing all age groups, including older people, and includes identifying:

- The severity and duration of previous disturbances
- The original and subsequent onset of symptoms
- Whether the patient has been hospitalized or treated by a psychiatrist
- Medication being received
- Successful past coping strategies or help
- Whether the patient is a suicide risk

Reminiscence therapy

The *Mosby Medical, Nursing and Allied Health Dictionary* (1994) defines reminiscence as the collection of past personal experiences and significant events. There are several functions of reminiscence therapy. It serves as self-therapy, an aid to gain new insight, a medium to put away troublesome events, and a way of rekindling lost skills or abilities (Edinberg, 1985). It is a psychotherapeutic technique in which self-esteem and personal satisfaction are restored by encouraging patients to review past experiences of a pleasant nature. Osborn (1990) states that reminiscence activities are frequently enjoyable and often energize older people, offering the opportunity to express a range of emotions such as sadness, anger, joy and frustration. In this way, many older people obtain considerable satisfaction from realizing that others feel that it is worth listening to stories of their lives.

Osborn (1990) also clarifies the characteristics of reminiscence as formal, informal, spontaneous, planned, verbal or activity-centred. A specific theme or focus is encouraged because it is more satisfying to remember details of events. Patients can select the theme themselves from a range of options such as childhood memories, family life, working years, relationships with others, and other specific life events. Various aids can be used to assist reminiscence including diaries, pictures, photographs, personal stories, books, poetry, slides, tapes, videos, music, objects and clothing. This can be facilitated by professionals, carers, other older people or children.

Coleman (1994) supports nurses and other professionals in using reminiscence because they are trained in listening and questioning skills, group facilitation skills, and the ability to manage conflict. Knowing a patient's past history is said to be beneficial, so that one is more able to empathize with that person. However, Osborn (1990) states that sadness does arise in reminiscence and that it is important not to be overprotective of people because they are old. It may be preferable to see patients individually if painful memories are expected. The provision of two facilitators for each group provides mutual support and greater opportunity to respond to individual patient's emotional needs. The size of a group is decided by the dependency levels of participants and the length of a session can vary between ten minutes and an hour, respecting that concentration spans vary between individuals.

Adams (1994) asserts that there is a danger if reminiscence provokes anger, unresolved grief, guilt or feelings of failure. A life review may include a range of results from nostalgia to severe depression and suicidal ideation, causing anxiety, guilt, despair and depression. Garland (1994) supports these concerns believing that the evaluation of life-review therapy is a matter for increasing concern. Negative outcomes are acknowledged but they do not appear in literature. This indicates to nurses who are facilitating reminiscence the need to assess the suitability of patients carefully before proceeding, to monitor the effects of therapy continually and discontinue it if it does not appear to be beneficial.

Bereavement therapy

Kubler-Ross (1969) identifies five stages of the grieving process. Although the original research by Kubler-Ross has been criticized because it focused only on women, the work is still universally accepted and specifies: denial and isolation, anger, bargaining, depression, and acceptance. The understanding is that a person experiencing death or loss encounters a period of bereavement. This is a natural rather than a pathological process. Depression is seen as part of this process. The process does not necessarily follow in sequence and it needs to be acknowledged that each individual's experience is unique.

Blazer (1993) proposes that medication should be avoided if possible. Respite should be temporary and new activities, relationships and independence in familiar surroundings should be encouraged.

Older people may have experienced many different types of loss in their lives, including that of: job, status and identity, income, health, confidence, and self-respect. Parkes (1990) provides a useful guide to risk factors that may highlight or predict those people who may be vulnerable to pathological grief. He suggests four main risk factors that may influence the bereavement process:

- Predisposing factors in the bereaved
- The relationship to the deceased
- The type of death
- The existing social support network

Social and environmental interventions

Normalization

The normalization process uses a multidisciplinary approach that places the patient at the centre of their own decision making and care planning. The focus is on assisting the individual to live as independently as possible, within a natural environment. This process was originally devised for people with learning disabilities (Wolfensberger, 1972). A key worker coordinates assessments from all relevant disciplines and brings the care team together for regular case conferences. The patient decides the number and priority of the needs that they wish to address. This is particularly appropriate for use with older people with depression, because it has a positive view of patients and validates them as individuals, improving their self-esteem. Normalization challenges the stigma of psychiatric nursing and ageism, which still exists in society and amongst some nurses (Walsh and Ford, 1989). Care plans are written using behavioural terms so that any multidisciplinary team member can easily identify and implement the care that has been agreed. Goals are broken down into a number of sequential steps, including a review date before progression to the next stage. By setting realistic goals jointly with a patient, care is more achievable and is reinforced positively.

A model of helping

When nursing an older person with depression, a nurse needs to consider what the appropriate approach is in order to manage care effectively. Jacobson and Makinnon (1989) outline a model of helping, which outlines six possible strategies that a nurse could choose:

- Giving information
- Taking action
- Giving advice
- Changing the system
- Teaching
- Counselling

The first five strategies assume that the helper has knowledge and awareness of the patient's needs. The strategies also encourage varying levels of dependence by the patient on the helper and are easier to use when a relationship has been established. The sixth strategy empowers the patient to take control and does not require for the helper to have all knowledge or recognize the needs of the patient, although a relationship is crucial to its success. It is useful for the nurse carefully to select the appropriate strategy for use with each patient according to specific needs and circumstances, and not to be influenced by his or her own preferred strategy of helping. However, it is beneficial for a nurse to acknowledge which strategies he or she may be most skilled at using, and those for which personal development and training are required.

Blazer (1993) states that an exhaustive comprehension of the literature related to the aetiology of later-life depression is not necessary for effective treatment. Multiple interventions, if orchestrated effectively, are even more likely to be successful. Most nurses would argue that they use a range of different types of helping strategies, which are determined by the individual needs of patients and their carers. It is crucial that nurses should consider the level of independence of the patient and are not guided by routine.

Family therapy

Rowe (1983) suggests that individuals create their own depression, but suggests that they can find a way out of their prison. She also believes that families can prevent this, particularly if the depression serves a function within the family system. Blazer (1993) suggests that the family needs to be evaluated, involving all family members as individuals. This includes reviewing the nuclear and extended family structure; the interactions and roles between members; the family atmosphere; family values; support systems and levels of tolerance; existing family stressors and family rewards. Treatment includes educating the family about depression; attempting to resolve any conflicts between family members; encouraging participation in the care of the depressed family member; and discussion of individual feelings. Many mental health nurses who are working in day hospitals and in the community develop valuable experience and skills by working with families and carers.

Humour therapy

There are many contrasting views of what constitutes humour. Some commentators refer to humour as situational jokes. Humour is a social lubricant, easing certain kinds of tension and shyness (Fry, 1963; Kubie, 1971; Pasquali, 1990). McDougal (1963) suggests that it is a behavioural response, which nature devised as an antidote to depression and pain. In contrast, Haig (1988) suggests that humour is a cognitive phenomenon, an intellectual process of perceiving and expressing what is amusing. Humour therapy is therefore about the constructive and therapeutic use of laughing with a person, and not a destructive use, characterized by laughing at others (Hillman, 1994). The response of an individual to humour can serve as a barometer and assessment to his or her internal states of anxiety and depression.

The literature supporting the use of humour is increasing in areas where people are vulnerable to depression, including counselling, psychotherapy and psychiatry (French, 1986; Haig, 1988; Mann, 1991). Mallet (1993) argues that limited clinical research has been conducted in the UK and advises that, at times, humour may be inappropriate and is best used with caution. If an older person is severely depressed, then humour may not be therapeutic and may merely serve to heighten the subject's awareness of how low his or her mood is. The subjective nature of humour requires that patients are assessed individually by the nurse for their level of suitability to different aspects of humour, accepting that a patient's mood may change during the day. Humour trolleys can be used containing humorous videos, audio cassettes, books, magazines, comics, poems, artwork, caricatures, games, puzzles and music (Mallett, 1995).

Massage therapy

Massage is a technique using a variety of hand strokes to move muscles and the soft tissues of the body. Benefits can be observed in the circulatory, lymphatic and nervous systems. Massage causes vasodilation of the peripheral circulation, resulting in a warming of the skin. Massaging towards lymph glands moves toxins away from the areas massaged. Sensory nerves are also stimulated, producing a relaxed response, including the benefits of touch (Maxwell-Hudson, 1988).

Fraser and Kerr (1993) report on the psychophysiological effects of back massage on elderly people in inpatient settings. Similarly, McKechnie et al. (1983) produced a report on the value of connective tissue massage in managing anxiety states. In this small study, individuals who were receiving massage either stopped or reduced the anxiolytics previously prescribed. It is interesting that, although nurses have shown great interest in massage within units for older people, limited literature is available demonstrating a commitment to this within mental health services for older people, where more research is clearly needed.

Essential oils

Essential oils are derived from flowers, leaves, seeds, wood, bark and roots of plants. Chemical analysis indicates the effects as being threefold. First, the pharmacological effect of essential oils is the reaction with hormones and enzymes in the body. Secondly, the physiological effect of these oils is in producing sedation and stimulation. Thirdly, there is the psychological effect of the aromas from the oils, which is considered very personal to each individual. Aromatherapy can be administered by massage (diluted in a cold-pressed oil of vegetable origin) vaporization, in baths, by compresses, and by spray (oil and water mixed). As with massage, the aspect of touch is an important feature of the therapy.

Passant (1990) showed that older patients in a ward environment and who were previously agitated, became much calmer following foot massage using essential oils. The use of lavender in a bath in the evening promoted restful sleep, resulting in the patients not requiring night sedation (Hewitt, 1992). There has been much research with essential oils in France (Tisserand, 1990), but this is limited in the UK.

Pet therapy

There is increasing interest in using pet therapy with older people, either by having a dog, a cat, a budgerigar or goldfish in wards and residential homes, or have them brought in by visiting friends, neighbours and carers.

Evaluating nursing intervention

Nurses need to evaluate the outcome of nursing interventions. Rawlins and Heacock (1993) provide a list of fourteen behaviours that would indicate a positive outcome of a nursing intervention. This list is useful when reflecting upon practice and monitoring standards of care. It is only by knowing and understanding a patient that a nurse is able to set realistic goals. A depressed patient who has responded positively to nursing interventions may:

- Be more animated
- Have more energy
- Eat nutritious meals regularly
- Sleep better
- Have no constipation
- Exercise regularly
- Include recreation in daily schedule
- Have fewer physical ailments
- Express feelings, both positive and negative
- Have less negative thinking
- Make positive statements about self and others
- Interact with others socially
- Be optimistic about the future
- Have a positive self-concept

Conclusion

Depression in old age is not part of the normal ageing process. It has been said that the classification of depression is carried out primarily by professionals, employing a medical model and scientific approach. This often differs from the experiences and perspectives of older people themselves. A variety of causes of depression in old age have been proposed. Different theories stress the influence of biophysical, social, environmental and psychological factors. These explanations provide a knowledge base from which nurses can gain a personal view of depression and select approaches to assessing and developing helping strategies for nursing older people.

The frequency of depression in older people appears difficult to determine, because they often present with an untypical picture of the illness. The features of depression are characterized by effects on an individual's emotional, physical, cognitive and social levels of functioning (Norman, 1991). Many older people therefore present with complex pictures and multiple pathologies, which can mask the symptoms of depression. This can lead to poor recognition and treatment. The larger numbers of older people, however, is likely to result in an increased incidence of depression in old age. It is therefore advantageous for nurses to be better informed and trained to assess this problem, using a variety of assessment methods.

Nurses working in hospital and community settings need to make it a priority to screen for depression and offer information and advice to patients regarding local resources and support networks for the maintenance of good mental health. Blazer (1993) advocates using a combined approach for the management of depression in older people. Nurses can use a range of skills, including counselling, cognitive behavioural, bereavement, reminiscence and family therapies. The effective management of physical illness and medication have equal importance, rather than being the main focus of attention. Nurses need to select interventions that are appropriate to their abilities and of relevance to the needs of older people as individuals.

Key points

- Nurses hold a key role in the assessment, care planning, monitoring and evaluation of nursing interventions and treatment of older people with depression.
- Nurses are in a key position to provide information and advice to individuals regarding possible preventive measures and the support that is available to older people with depression.
- Nurses need to be aware of their own values and beliefs about depression and the influence that these have on their approach to nursing.
- Nurses need to work in collaboration with other health care professionals and initiate mechanisms that encourage a consistent approach to care.
- Nurses have the choice of selecting from different helping strategies and nursing interventions, to provide flexible practice.
- Nurses need to be mindful individually of their abilities and limitations when nursing older people with depression.
- Nurses are individually responsible for developing their practice and ensuring that they have adequate support for themselves.
- Nurses as a group need to undertake more research to test and discover more creative and innovative therapeutic interventions for nursing older people with depression.

References

Adams, J. (1994). A fair hearing: life-review in a hospital setting. In *Reminiscence Reviewed: Rethinking Ageing.* (J. Bornat, ed.) pp. ?. Buckingham: Open University Press.

Beaumont. G. and Anfield, E. (1983). Suicide and Depression: Risk and Prevention. *Psychiatry Pract.* Proceedings of a symposium held at University Hospital of South Manchester, West Didsbury, Manchester, 19 January.

Beck, A. T. (1976). *Cognitive Therapy and the Emotional Disorders.* New York: International Universities Press.

Beck, A. T., Ward, C. H., Mendelson, M. et al. (1961). An inventory for measuring depression. *Arch. Gen. Psychiatry,* **4**, 561–571.

Beck, A. T., Rush, A. J., Shaw, B. F. and Emery, G. (1979). *Cognitive Therapy of Depression.* New York: Wiley.

Beck, C., Modlin, T., Heithoff, K. and Shue, V. (1992). Exercise as an intervention for behaviour problems. *Geriatr. Nurs.,* **13**, 273–275.

Benbow. S. M. (1991). Old age psychiatrists' view of the use of ECT. *Int. J. Geriatr. Psychiatry,* **6**, 317–322.

Blazer, D. G. (1993). *Depression in Late Life,* 2nd ed. St. Louis, MO: Mosby.

British Association for Counselling. (1984). *Code of Ethics.* Rugby: BAC.

British Association for Counselling. (1989). *Definition of Counselling.* Rugby: BAC.

Case-McAleer, D. (1993). Highstepping exercise program promotes strength; self esteem. *Provider,* **19**(1) 47.

Coleman, P. (1994). Reminiscence within the study of ageing: the social significance of story. In: *Reminiscence Reviewed: Rethinking Ageing.* (J. Bornat, ed.) pp. 8–20, Buckingham: Open University Press.

Dryden, W. (1989). The use of chaining in rational emotive therapy. *J. Rational Emotive Ther.,* **7**, 59–66

Dzyak, J. M. (1990). *An investigation of the effects of an exercise on joint range of motion on healthy females, 62 years of age or older.* Boston, MA: Boston University. DNSC.

Edinberg, M. A. (1985). *Mental Health Practice with the Elderly.* Englewood Cliffs, NJ: Prentice Hall.

Egan, G. (1994). *The Skilled Helper: a Problem Management Approach in Helping.* 5th ed. Pacific Grove, CA: Brooks Cole.

Ellgring, H. (1989). *Non-Verbal Communication in Depression.* (European Monographs in Social Psychology). Cambridge: Cambridge University Press.

Fraser, J. and Kerr, J. R. (1993). Psychological effects of back massage on elderly institutionalised patients. *J. Adv. Nurs.,* **18**, 238–245.

French, J. (1986). Health Education. Don't make me laugh. *J. Inst. Health Educ.,* **24**(2), 53–59.

Fry, W. F. (1963). *Sweet Madness. A Study of Humour.* Palo Alto CA: Pacific Books.

Garland, J. (1994). What splendour, it all coheres: life-review therapy with older people. In: *Reminiscence Reviewed: Rethinking Ageing.* (J. Bornat, ed.) pp. 21–31, Buckingham: Open University Press.

Gearing, B., Johnson, M. and Heller, T. (1988). *Mental Health Problems in Old Age.* (A Wiley Medical Publication in association with The Open University.) Chichester: Wiley.

Gilbert, P. (1992). *Counselling for Depression: Counselling in Practice.* London: Sage.

Haig, R. A. (1988). Some socio-cultural aspects of humour. *Aust. N. Z. J. Psychiatry*, **22**, 418–422.

Healy, D. (1993). *Psychiatric Drugs Explained*. London: Mosby Year Book.

Hewitt, D. (1992). Massage with lavender oil lowered tension. *Nurs. Times*, **88**(25), 8.

Hillman, S. (1994). The healing power of humour at work. *Nurs. Stand.*, **8**(42), 31–34.

Holmes, T. H. and Rahe, R. H. (1967). The social readjustment rating scale. *J. Psychosom. Res.*, **11**, 213–218.

Jacobs, M. (1988). *Psychodynamic Counselling in Action.* (Counselling In Action Series.) London: Sage.

Jacobson, F. and Makinnon, H. (1989). *Sharing Counselling Skills: a Guide to Running Courses for Nurses, Midwives and Health Visitors*. Edinburgh: Scottish Health Education Group.

Kendell, R. D. (1976). The classification of depression: a review of contemporary confusion. *Br. J. Psychiatry.*, **129**, 15–28.

Kubie, L. S. (1971). The destructive potential of humour in psychotherapy. *Am. J. Psychiatry*, **127**(7), 37–42.

Kubler-Ross, E. (1969). *On Death and Dying*. London: Routledge.

Mallet, J. (1993). Use of humour and laughter in patient care. *Br. J. Nurs.*, **2**, 172–175.

Mallet, J. (1995). Humour and laughter therapy. *Complementary Ther. Nurs. Midwifery*, **1**, 73–76.

Mann, D. (1991). Humour in psychotherapy. *Psychoanal. Psychother.*, **5**, 161–170.

Maxwell-Hudson, C. (1988). *The Complete Book of Massage*. London: Dorling Kindersley.

McDougal, W. (1963). *An Instinct of Laughter, an Introduction to Social Psychology.* New York: Unison Paperbacks.

McKechnie, A. A., Wilson, F., Watson, N. and Scott, D. (1983). Anxiety states: a preliminary report on the value of connective tissue masage. *J. Psychosom. Res.*, **27**, 125–129.

Mosby Medical, Nursing and Allied Health Dictionary, 4th ed. (1994). St Louis, MO: Mosby.

Murphy, E (1982). Social origins of depression in old age. *Br. J. Psychiatry*, **141**, 135–142.

Murphy, E., Lindsay, J. and Grundy, E. (1986). Sixty years of suicide in England and Wales. *Arch. Gen. Psychiatry*, **43**, 969–977.

Murphy, G. E., Simons, A. D., Wetzel, R. D. and Lustman, P. J. (1984). Cognitive therapy and pharmacotherapy: singly and together in the treatment of depression. *Arch. Gen. Psychiatry*, **41**, 33–41

Nelson-Jones, R. (1993). *Practical Counselling and Helping Skills*, 3rd ed. London: Cassell.

Norman, I. J. (1991). Depression in old age. In *Nursing Elderly People*, (S. J. Redfern, ed.), pp. 341–372. London: Churchill Livingstone.

Osborn, C. (1990). *A Practical Guide to Reminiscence Work*. London: Age Exchange.

Parkes, C. M. (1990). Risk factors in bereavement: implications for the prevention and treatment of pathologic grief. *Psychiatr. Ann.*, **20**, 308–313

Pasquali, E. A. (1990). Learning to laugh: humour as therapy. *J. Psychosoc. Nurs. Ment. Health Serv.* **28**(3), 31–35.

Passant, H. (1990). A holistic approach in the ward. *Nurs. Times*, **86**(4), 26–28.

Pitt, B. (1988). Characteristics of depression in the elderly. In *Mental Health Problems in Old Age*. (A Wiley Medical Publication in association with The Open University.) (B. Gearing, M. Johnson and T. Heller, eds.) pp. 114–122. Chichester: Wiley. 114-122.

Pleuvry, B. J. and Snowdon, A. T. (1988). *The Nurse, Drugs and the Patient*. Oxford: Blackwell Scientific.

Post, F. (1981). Affective illnesses. In *Health Care of the Elderly*. (T. Arie, ed.) pp. 89–103. London: Croom Helm.

Rawlins, R. P. and Heacock, P. E. (1993). *Clinical Manual of Psychiatric Nursing*. 2nd ed. London: Mosby Year Book.

Rowe, D. (1983). *Depression: The Way Out of Your Prison*. London: Routledge.

Royal College of Nursing. (1990). *Guidelines for Assessment of Elderly People*. London: RCN.

Scrutton, S. (1989). *Counselling Older People. A Creative Response to Ageing*. (Age Concern Handbooks). London: Edward Arnold.

Seligman, M. E. (1975). *Helplessness*. San Francisco, CA: Freeman.

Sheehan, A. (1994). Extending the role of mental health nurses. *Nurs. Stand.*, **8**(44), 31–34.

Tisserand, R. (1990). Aromatherapy for everyone. London: Akana.

Topp, R. (1991). Development of an exercise program for older adults: pre-exercise testing, exercise precription and program maintenance. *Nurse Pract. (Am. J. Primary Health Care)*, **16**(10), 16–18, 20–21, 25–26.

Walsh, M. and Ford, P. (1989). *Nursing Rituals: Research and Rational Actions*. Oxford: Butterworth-Heinemann.

Weinstein, L. B. (1986). The benefits of aquatic activity. *J. Gerontol. Nurs.*, **12**(2), 6–11.

Wilkinson, G. (1989). *Depression*. (Family Doctor Guides Series). London: British Medical Association.

Williams, J. M. G. (1992). *The Psychological Treatment of Depression: a Guide to the Theory and Practice of Cognitive Behavioural Therapy*. London: Routledge.

Wolfensberger, W. (1972). *The Principle of Normalisation in Human Services*. Toronto: The National Institute on Mental Retardation.

8

Challenging behaviour

Niall Grant
Dedicated to the memory of Marjory Irving

Introduction

Aim pridem Syrus in Tiberim defluxit Orontes Et linguam et mores
                                                    Juvenal *c*.60 to *c*.130 AD

(The Syrian Orontes has now for long been pouring into the Tiber, with its own language and ways of behaving.)

Challenging behaviour in older people with mental health problems is no new phenomenon. People of all ages, not unlike the Syrian Orontes, can challenge and demonstrate, through their behaviour. Challenging behaviour is not an exclusive symptom of increasing age or illness; it is a method by which we make our thoughts and feelings known. The interpretation of the behaviour as 'challenging' may well highlight the observer's viewpoint and not accurately define the behaviour observed. Thus, challenging behaviour could be described as 'any behaviour that has a negative effect on the individual or others'.

When an elderly person with mental health problems demonstrates in a manner that is not acceptable to the social norm, the first response should be to ask why this is happening:

- Why are they acting in such a way?
- Why are they doing it now?
- Have they done this before?
- How often does it occur? How long does it last? Does its intensity vary?
- How have my actions affected this?
- How effective have previous interventions been, and why?
- What interventions are available that will not reduce the quality of life?

Challenging behaviour can be viewed using its component parts:

- *Antecedent:* what caused the behaviour?
- *Behaviour:* the behaviour is observed as challenging
- *Consequence:* what is the outcome of the behaviour?

The ability to analyse challenging behaviour as a three-stage entity enables easier assessment, planning, implementation and evaluation. There is no directory of interventions available, each behaviour is as unique as the individual exhibiting it.

The key to more defined nursing intervention is based on a thorough knowledge of the person, the nurse's abilities to observe, and motivation to reduce the cause(s) of the challenging behaviour.

Challenging behaviour does not fit neatly into a procedural pigeonhole. There are no standard signs and symptoms. It may be in response to:

- Physical illness: cerebrovascular accident, infections
- Mental illness: depression, anxiety, psychosis
- Pain
- Environment: home, light, sounds, temperature, changes
- Sensory loss: reduced visual acuity, hearing, taste, smell or touch
- Medication side effects
- Alcohol and drug abuse and misuse
- Anger, boredom and frustration

To commence an effective analysis of and intervention in challenging behaviour requires the resolution to do so, and the acceptance that there are often options to previous practices. There is no doubt in my mind that the single most effective intervention in any challenging behaviour is a skilled nursing team applying planned nursing care. Medication, when clinically indicated, may help, but total dependence on the administration of benzodiazepines, phenothiazines and butyrophenones is an easy way out and should be seen as a last resort.

Aim

The aim of this chapter is not to provide prescriptive interventions for every incident of challenging behaviour, but rather to encourage readers to examine their understanding of and their response to challenging behaviour, and to assist nurses individually to apply their skills to greater effect, thus improving the quality of care for their patients/clients/residents.

Within this chapter the main issues for the nurse to revisit are:

- Defining what is challenging behaviour
- Examining their response (and the response of others) to challenging behaviour
- Using the nursing process to aid their programme of care
- Examining the needs of patients as individuals and as a group, and of their carers, and examining the nursing role

Rationale/background

New areas for many nurses are the structured observation of individuals with challenging behaviour, the meaningful management of this behaviour and the devising of a structured plan of care that can measure its reduction. What is most testing of all is that this process should be readily understood by all those who participate in the care of these individuals.

The successful nursing of challenging behaviour in older people with mental health problems is an area of immense importance. By choosing not to recognize challenging behaviour as a possible symptom of the less obvious, nurses elect to ignore individuality and the need for specific care planning. They choose to dismiss causes of challenging behaviour, such as possible side effects of medication, disorientation because of illness itself, or underlying infection or physiological disease processes. The unwillingness to see each person as a dynamic individual who is capable of change creates a self-fulfilling prophecy.

Challenging behaviour in older people has been long neglected and now requires to be redressed as a specialty skill in its own right. Nurses who are capable of achieving a successful reduction in challenging behaviour within an institutional setting (hospital or residential) can provide extra skills for those carers and community staff who are dealing with challenging behaviour in a home setting.

Literature review

A literature review shows that there are reasons why the recognition, definition and effective care of challenging behaviour in older people is required. It appears from my experience that behaviours have been seen historically as purely symptomatic of illness, treated with medication, or poorly tolerated.

It may be that the care of older people is not viewed positively, and that the structure of nursing work with inflexible routines that are focused on physical care, and also the high dependency needs of some elderly people, makes this area of nursing less glamorous as a career choice (Pursey and Luker, 1995). There has been a growing awareness of the need to address challenging behaviour in elderly mentally ill people as an evidence-based skill. Similar needs have been developed in the field of learning disabilities and there are obvious areas of transferable skills between the two (Tarbuck and Thompson, 1995). Historically, challenging behaviours were referred to as 'problem' behaviours. This focused on the patient as having the problem. By defining the behaviour as 'challenging', the emphasis is less directed towards the patient's problem, but rather towards the environment in which the behaviour was shown (Darbyshire and Whitaker, 1990). Thus, this move of the emphasis away from the negative may well make the need to meet the challenge more positive (i.e. the enhancement of individual care through met needs and wants).

The incidence of challenging behaviour may well be a matter of interpretation. Rossby et al. (1992) define 'disruptive' behaviour as 'behaviour which has negative consequences for the resident, caregiver, or other residents'. Thus, there is a need to identify and more finely tune the definition of which behaviours are challenging. Byrne (1994) noted that 'the nature of these behaviours [physical aggression and screaming] is such that they are unlikely to be tolerated for long, even in the most sympathetic surroundings and by the most sympathetic observers'. Consequently, there is a need to identify which behaviours are challenging, and to whom. In a review of the literature on disruptive behaviour in older people, Beck et al. (1997) noted that the impact on patients and staff can include stress, decreased quality of care, injuries to staff, absenteeism, staff burnout, increased staff turnover, social isolation of disruptive patients, and ironically, an increased occurrence of falls and injury. They also composed a list of forty-five disruptive behaviours, ranging from 'inappropriate ambulation' to 'use of a weapon'. There is also a deficit in the instruments used to define and measure challenging behaviour. The Revised Elderly Persons Disability Scale will identify behaviour likely to require an increased proactive nursing response, but does not allow for the day-to-day, and hour-to-hour measurement of behaviour and the impact of intervention. Historically, nurses have relied on anecdotal or subjective measurements, which can lead to value judgements and inaccuracy in defining, planning, implementing and measuring the success of planned care. Again, Beck et al. (1997) noted in their study of developing and testing an instrument to assess the severity of disruptive behaviour in older people with mental health problems, that nurses were capable of accurately defining and recording disruptive behaviour in their patients. Structured intervention can be influenced greatly by a nurse's favoured approach.

Followers of the method of validation therapy (Feil, 1992) or of reality orientation (Holden, 1995) may well adopt a correct approach, but be inaccurate in their measurement of outcomes.

Finally, a complete faith in drug administration as the primary intervention is flawed for the following reasons. Benzodiazepines can be highly addictive, butyrophenones and phenothiazines have unpleasant side effects in older people. They can all mask an individual's needs and, ultimately, reduce quality of life through prolonging the unmet need that originally caused the prescription of the medication. In a study of the misprescription of inappropriate tranquillizers and antipsychotic drugs, McGrath and Jackson (1996) cited the controls placed on American doctors in the treatment of challenging behaviour in older people. A redefinition of symptoms and appropriate drug treatment prevented the prescribing of inappropriate drugs. If this was to be enforced in the UK, nurses would have to rethink the archaic practices surrounding management of challenging behaviour. The administration of neuroleptic medication, as noted by McShane et al. (1997), may worsen already poor cognitive function in dementia.

The subject matter

Before moving on, there are several important principles to follow, which should not only help the reader in structuring care but also assist in structuring a staff team approach to the philosophy of care and better prepare staff for the work ahead.

Is there a defined clinical leader who can coordinate and facilitate the changes needed?

A disjointed and noncohesive team will not function, and older people's needs will not be met and sustained. A team leader must be identified. This is essential in coordinating practice, whether it is based on the care needs of one individual patient or, as happens more often, of a group of patients/ clients/residents who present a range of challenging behaviours.

Know the person!

To understand and know the older person is an obvious requirement, but this is ritually ignored. The resources to hand, excluding the patient's own account, are varied. Biographies, life stories and medical histories are essential, as is identification of the ways in which families and carers can help. Often, the challenging behaviour that you witness causes the family great concern and embarrassment, and may have done so before admission of the older person to the clinical area.

Create a culture of change

Question: How do you eat an elephant?

Answer: In small bites over a long period

Undoubtedly, things will have to change if you earnestly wish to nurse challenging behaviour successfully. Scenarios that feature the intransigent registered nurse and the ogre of a nursing assistant working together to undermine any procedure being done other than in the way it has always been done, are sadly still alive and kicking.

The team leader must be strong enough to share his or her vision with conviction and not expect miracles overnight. However, a philosophy of care that espouses the importance of defining patient needs and wants accurately, and promotes proactive nursing care and staff development, is a good starting point.

Aims must be realistic and resources identified

Nurses must be realistic in their aims, and define short-, medium- and long-term goals. They must identify the available resources, both human and other. As an example, consider a vision to create an environment that is conducive to living, visiting and working, which is nonthreatening and acknowledges the individual's needs.

Look at your work area. Would you like to live here? Does it offer you privacy, allow dignity, and provide places to be alone and to be in the company of those you choose? Do the staff listen to you, talk over you, ignore you, attempt to understand you? Does it smell pleasant, sound therapeutic and look inviting, or are their three competing sources of TV, radio, etc? Are there glaring strip lights or windows without curtains or blinds? These are just a few of the questions you might want to ask, including the essential: 'Am I given the opportunity to choose, to discuss and refuse'?

If you are of the opinion that your place of work does not offer the above then you may have stumbled on the answer to some of the causes of challenging behaviour.

Rigid inflexible routines can account for some demonstrative behaviour, although not all

How honest are you? If you lived in your work environment, would your colleagues know all your idiosyncracies? Would they attempt to learn some of them? Do they know that some days you are hungrier than others, that your sleep pattern fluctuates, or that your feelings reflect your need for company. If your colleagues were to glean this information, how would they do it? How accurate is their method of documentation? Does it read like a bowel chart and bathing timetable? Do your colleagues have a clear idea of the physiological changes associated with advancing age? Are they familiar with the less speedy responses to the demands of your major body systems?

In short, are you in a culture that recognizes the need to adapt and change, a culture that recognizes its shortfalls, and is willing to address them? It is often very easy to spot the environmental impact on behaviour when you visit somewhere for the first time. Oh for the halcyon days of carbolic smelling linoleum, the solid click of sensible brogues and the efficient rustle of heavily starched uniforms. Not a bowel movement out of sync!

Ask a friendly 'other' or a new member of staff, or one returning from holiday, to visit your clinical area with a critical eye. Take note and look at the way in which nurses skilfully and unintentionally erode the homeliness of the area. Obviously, the area has a clinical obligation, but this need not exclude warmth or a pleasant ambience. This sleuthing approach will also highlight nurses' ability to ignore privacy and dignity.

By this stage, perhaps, the reader has had a few twinges of professional guilt. As an example of the impact of environment on challenging behaviour, try experimenting with the lighting in your area. At night, reduce the lighting in a brightly lit area by using small table lamps instead of strip lights; create light pockets with small groups of chairs, coffee tables, etc. Monitor the degree of patient traffic pacing or wandering the previously overlit areas. It should reduce as people find their corner. Make a small feature of a television, radio or hi-fi system. Interactions with individuals will become easier and more personal.

It is wise also to remember the basic principles of nursing: remaining calm and not being confrontational, treating the individual patient as a person, promoting patient choice, and communicating with others, especially making time for reflective practice.

Defining and recognizing challenging behaviour

In defining challenging behaviour, it is important to look at your own definition or previous examples of challenging behaviour. Ultimately, you will become aware that a divergence from the social norms of the prevailing culture has occurred. In extreme cases, this may involve bodily harm to carers or to individual patients/clients. However, breaches of social norms may entail nonconforming to the expected decorum, and lead to the marginalizing of an individual.

Vignette 1

Jonathan, a retired bank manager, has a moderate degree of dementia and now lives in a nursing home due to the increased demands of care on his elderly wife. The home caters specifically for those with dementia. A problem, however, has arisen. Jonathan has started to pace the corridors, pull buttons off his shirts and cardigans, and is now walking out of the refectory-style dining room at lunch and dinner times.

Staff are fearful that he may become aggressive, especially when out in public. The GP has prescribed diazepam, and Jonathan dozes for much of the day. The fear of verbally aggressive outbursts comes true when staff attempt to coerce Jonathan into eating in the dining room. Unfortunately, the staff can take no more and Jonathan is admitted to a psychiatric hospital. On his admission, his wife is concerned that her husband will cause problems and is obviously embarrassed by his behaviour. In order to assess him and his behaviour, staff took a detailed history, quickly learning that Jonathan has never enjoyed sitting with large groups of people. His button-tearing happened during lunch and dinner times, or for an hour or so afterwards. He always ate a hearty breakfast in his bedroom in the nursing home.

The information gained came mostly from Jonathan's wife and through observation of his behaviour. Needless to say, meals were offered in his room or, as it became his favourite, in a small sitting room with three other men. The button-tearing stopped. The diazepam was reduced over time to preclude possible withdrawal effects. No verbal or physical aggression was observed, and this quiet man spent much time reading his golf magazines and participating in small group activities.

Could his button tearing have been due to anxiety or frustration as a result of sitting in a large, noisy area?

In recounting Jonathan's case, several important points were raised. There was an obvious inability of the nursing home staff to see that their expectations of Jonathan were not realistic; his wife had not been consulted about his life style, and the staff were unable to admit that they were creating a self-fulfilling prophecy by not examining their role in nursing Jonathan.

The methods of assessment were not complex and the reduction in Jonathan's challenging behaviour was accomplished easily, without resorting to detailed documentation and observation. It was also economical because it involved ward-based staff who were prepared to observe and accept this man as unique. The culture of the psychiatric ward was to accept individuals as such. By reducing the frustration felt and expressed by Jonathan, it can be assumed that he felt a little happier in himself.

Not all instances of challenging behaviour are so easily assessed and resolved. The principles remain the same; that is, to assess and observe, and to plan, implement and evaluate. In the next clinical example, a greater degree of observation and interpretation of findings was required, especially a critical review of the assumptions of the multidisciplinary team.

Vignette 2

Carolyn, an eighty-five-year-old lady with severe dementia and limited vocabulary, who was nonweight-bearing, chair shaped with contractures and grossly underweight according to standardized dietetic charts, presented a challenge to the nursing and dietetic staff: Carolyn refused to eat, invariably spitting out what food the nursing staff attempted to give her.

Due to her low body weight, the dieticians commenced her on a high protein diet, which included liquid and semiliquid supplements. The nursing staff adopted a novel way of ensuring that Carolyn's nutritional intake had a greater rate of success, which was by squirting the liquidized diet into her mouth through large syringes.

This scenario is not productive. It was obvious that Carolyn was communicating something; her behav·our said so. The nursing staff, although well intentioned, were ignoring her basic human rights and endangering her through the increased risk of aspiration pneumonia.

Nursing staff reassessed this challenging behaviour:

- Why did Carolyn spit out the food?
- Did it taste awful?
- Was she given too much?
- Was she objecting to the method, frequency and speed at which she was fed?

- Did she have any choice in the matter; was she hungry?
- The list of questions went on . . .

The action taken was to:

- Assess Carolyn's appetite versus her need to eat
- Assess the quality, quantity and choice of food
- Assess the meal times; were they suitable for Carolyn?
- Assess the eating environment
- Assess the staff motives: their needs versus Carolyn's

Outcome

Carolyn's nutritional intake was in fact adequate for her. A detailed study was made of Carolyn's eating patterns, the eating environment, the time of day, and the quality and quantity of food that she actually ate. It involved the monitoring of her weight and, conceivably, other activities of living. These observations of her eating pattern and preferences showed that she tended to enjoy larger meals every second day, without a further significant reduction in her body mass and weight. Snacks and drinks were more enthusiastically taken. There was a vast reduction in the spitting out of food and an increase in the amount of time staff spent with Carolyn and other patients in small lunch group-type settings.

Was her apparent satisfaction with her diet reflected in improved sleep and her ability to socialize? The staff realized that other patients might have similar needs/wants and became more attuned to this possibility.

This example of charting and monitoring the challenging behaviour involved more than a review of the notes. It included the questioning of staff attitudes to dietary needs, and staff (unwittingly) impinging on their patients' wants.

The final scenario involved detailed measurement of the presenting baseline behaviour including its frequency and intensity, and environmental factors (including individual staff members), follow-up measurements, and an ongoing evaluation of implemented care.

Vignette 3

Danny, a sixty-seven-year-old man with Korsakoff's disease, had further neurological damage due to cerebral anoxia following cardiopulmonary resuscitation. He was nonweight-bearing and completely dependent on staff for washing, dressing and eating. His behavioural response to staff and peer interactions was unpredictably violent, often with biting and scratching and screaming abuse at staff.

Many staff were fearful of him and reluctant to engage in any meaningful interactions. The nursing response was to limit interactions and rely heavily on phenothiazines to reduce his aggressive outbursts. The result was that Danny was successfully ignored and isolated, and there was a dramatic reduction in his self-care skills and (arguably) his quality of life.

Table 8.1 Incidence of assault on and abuse of staff

Day/Time	Male staff	Female staff	Biting	Scratching	Shouting	In bed	Chair	Bedroom	Living-room	Incont: faeces	Incont: urine
1	•		+	+	+	•		•			++
2		•	+++	+	+	•		•			
3	•		+	++	++		•		•		+
4		•		+++	+++		•		•		
5	•	•	+++	++	++	•		•		++	++

• an incident
+ amount of assault/abuse relative to the heading

First, (auto)biographical information from Danny, his siblings and his partner was gathered to gauge his preferences, needs and wants. Structured baseline observations of Danny's behaviour were carried out, together with a review of all his aggressive/violent incidents, the environment in which they occurred, the time of day, the staff who were in attendance, etc. When possible, antecedants, behaviours and consequences were identified. A cluster chart was used to summarize the incidents and variables involved. Table 8.1 gives a short sample summary of the results obtained by charting Danny's behaviour, and collating its frequency, intensity and other environmental variables. This is merely a snapshot of much day-by-day note taking; however an early trend did develop. Male staff were less likely to be assaulted on their own than were female staff. The intensity of Danny's verbal and physical abuse was greatest when he was incontinent of faeces. He was more inclined to assault if woken by staff rather than when he awoke without prompting. Day-shift staff were more likely to be assaulted than night-shift staff. What the chart does not indicate is the fact that Danny had a more positive response to specific staff. It was through the development of these relationships that Danny's behavioural programme was explained to him and implemented.

This included standardized verbal responses to Danny's assaults by all staff, including the choice for Danny to accept or refuse staff interaction. Staff used a calm and nonjudgemental approach, and would inform Danny of their sadness at his need to respond violently during their interactions with him.

Danny had the choice to have male staff nurse him when possible. If this was not possible, an explanation was given. His opinion on his choice of clothing, the style of his beard and the mirror in which to watch himself being shaved was sought.

The outcome, although ongoing, was a marked reduction in his physical aggression towards staff and his peers, even during washing him after faecal incontinence, which had usually provoked his potentially most violent episodes. Danny became a man whom staff sought out rather than avoided or feared. Other emotional responses became evident and he was witnessed laughing and crying appropriately. With Jonathan, he chose the wine for small lunch parties.

These examples are based on real nursing interventions. They are, however, purely a summary, and do not reflect the hard work involved by all grades of nurses in the clinical team, or the wide range of conditions that might produce challenging behaviour. An individual with challenging behaviour as a result of a depressive illness will hopefully show a decrease in symptoms as the depression lifts and may require adaptation of the intervention. This still indicates the need for nurses to meet challenging behaviour in a knowledgeable and structured way, basing each patient's care on individual needs and wants.

Summary

If nurses wish to develop care for older people with mental health problems, and if they wish to be seen as proactive and capable, then addressing the subject of challenging behaviour is essential. The principles discussed above are just that, principles. It is the individual needs of the patient, whether at home or in an institutional setting, that must be both the bottom and top lines for care provision. The need for staff training and development with the acquisition of specialist skills in this area, is paramount. Consequently, the onus falls on the individual with motivation as well as, in a broader sense, the profession and employers. If the drug prescription laws that prevail in the USA were to be enforced in the UK, the need to re-examine effective nursing care might be rushed into with little forethought or individual patient planning.

The methods by which challenging behaviour can be handled by nurses are not new. The need to break inflexible routines is not new. The need to use the nursing process in this situation is not new. The need to educate ourselves and colleagues is not new. Nurses are more than capable of objectively observing, designing and implementing care to a high standard.

Ultimately, there is a need to elucidate a standardized definition of challenging behaviour in older people who have mental health problems, and to delineate effective strategies to implement their care, but the basic requirement is the motivation to provide accurately targeted care for individuals.

References

Beck, C., Heithoff, K., Baldwin, B., Cuffel, B., O Sullivan, P. and Chumbles, N. (1997). Assessing disruptive behaviour in older adults: the disruptive behaviour scale. *Aging Ment. Health*, **1**, 71–79.

Byrne, E. J. (1994). *The management of confusional states in older people*. London: Edward Arnold.

Darbyshire, P. and Whitaker, S. (1990). The final challenge. *Nurs. Times*, **86**(2), 64–65.

Feil, N. (1992). Validation: the Feil method: how to help the disoriented old. Cleveland, Ohio: Edward Feil Productions.

Holden, U. (1995). Ageing, neuropsychology and the 'new' dementias: definitions, explanations and practical approaches. London: Chapman and Hall.

Mcgrath, A. M. and Jackson, G. J. (1996). Survey of neuroleptic prescribing in residents of nursing homes in Glasgow. *Br. Med. J.*, **312**, 611–612.

McShane, R. (1997). Do neuroleptic drugs hasten cognitive decline in dementia? Prospective study with necropsy follow up. *Br. Med. J.*, **314**, 266–270.

Pursey, A. and Luker, K. (1995). Attitudes and stereotypes: nurses' work with older people. *J. Adv. Nurs.*, **22**, 547–555.

Rossby, L., Beck, C. and Heacock, P. (1992). Disruptive behaviours of cognitively impaired nursing home residents. *Arch. Psychiatr. Nurs.*, **6**, 98–107.

Tarbuck, P. and Thompson, A. (1995). Defining and treating challenging behaviour. *Nurs. Stand.*, **9**(42), 30–33.

9

Dealing with Dilemmas

Alan Crump

Introduction

This chapter provides an insight into some of the ethical and moral implications of caring for older people's mental health needs. Ageism and wider social and political issues will be discussed, which will be the backdrop to the chapter. It will consider issues related to the rights of older people with mental illness and will tackle the difficult issue of risk taking. There will be a section on the problem of the abuse of older people, which is of increasing concern.

The points will be discussed in a style that will encourage the reader towards further thought and analysis. They will be relevant to those who work in hospitals and in the community, whether in an individual's home or in nursing homes. It is intended to study past practice, highlight current good practice and point the direction for future practice.

The aim of this chapter is to provide the reader with the opportunity to explore some of the practice dilemmas, ethical issues and moral implications of nursing care.

Myths and stereotypes

Older people in our society are disadvantaged by attitudes that reduce them to a group with minority status. Society has tended to label older people as either the very vulnerable or the completely extraordinary. The same newspaper will print a story about a frail pensioner too frightened to go outside, while in the same issue portray the sprightly great-grandfather who has just gained his Open University degree (Midwinter, 1988). The effect of this stereotyping is to box older people into certain groups; like the frail old lady; the robust and proud old soldier; the eccentric old spinster; the academic older tutor; or the confused and perplexed old man. This need to put older people into particular groups serves only to marginalize these individuals still further (Norman, 1987a). Despite this wish to classify people into groups and sections, it remains to be truly accepted that there is no all-embracing group of the over sixty-fives, just as there is no average teenager. To suggest that, on receiving a pension, older people conform to a homogeneous state, is to believe that a lifetime of experience has not coloured the hopes and aspirations of a diverse population of people who find themselves over the age of sixty-five years.

The end of an established money-earning capacity does not denote the loss of individuality or of personality. People who retire from paid employment usually develop a myriad of interests and activities that reflect their individual preferences and life style. This will be influenced by their previous life style and the pensions and savings they may have at their disposal. Retired older people do not become a uniform group with the same values and beliefs. It is likely that the values that they hold once they have retired will be a reflection of those held while they were working. An individual's politics do not change overnight because they have retired, just as a regular attender at a place of worship does not suddenly lose their faith. The avid sports devotee does not lose the passion for sport or an environmentalist lose the drive to campaign. However, these values and beliefs may alter in retirement, with reflection, just as they alter and develop throughout our entire lives.

For some, the age of 'retirement' does not lead to a reduced money-earning capacity. For those in politics, the law, medicine or the arts, or who are members of a church, age does not denote a time for reduced prestige and loss of status. There is, instead, a sense of enhanced respect for accumulated knowledge and, in these fields, individuals are encouraged to continue their work. Long service can be valued positively and there may be only a modest loss of earnings. However, the real benefit is the continued status that accompanies employment (Stokes, 1992).

There are also significant numbers of people who, after retirement, find part-time work and continue to play an active part in the workplace. This may not carry with it the status and financial security that full-time employment brought, but it creates some of the structure that a full-time post offers. However, great value is placed upon the capacity to earn money and the age of retiring carries with it many negative connotations. There are advertisements for certain employment areas that ask for applicants of a certain (younger) age, openly discriminating against older workers. There are few guidelines to protect against this particularly blatant discrimination and the loss of work rights of older persons. To those who find themselves out of work through retirement or redundancy in their later years, it can be an uphill struggle to find work. Overnight, one's position in a society that favours productivity and money-earning capacity can start to move on a downward course.

Older people are not the only group in society to suffer from discrimination. It is common in many groups, as a result of colour, culture, gender, sexuality or nationality. A large group for whom discrimination is an everyday event are those with mental health needs. For any of us, the sight of someone in the street who is exhibiting bizarre behaviour, or who is dressed very unusually, is likely to bring about uneasy feelings and a tendency to avoid that person. It is only recently that efforts have been made properly to integrate and rehabilitate people with mental health needs into everyday environments (Department of Health, 1990). In the past, people were offered protection in large asylums, far from the sensitive eyes of 'normal' people. The efforts to bring about care in the community have made moves to break down these negative stereotypes, but there remains a desperate need to forge a more positive image of people who have mental health problems.

This leaves older people with a mental illness in a doubly disadvantaged position (Norman, 1982). If one adds to this the stigma attached to one of the chronic mental health problems, that of dementia, then the picture becomes ever more blurred and stigmatized. The poor understanding of dementia, and also the great fear attached to having dementia, only add to the stigma. Such is the misconception regarding dementia that it is assumed by many to be the major mental health issue for older people, when, in fact, it is easily outstripped by depression (Brayne and Ames, 1988). This image was reflected in a series of newspaper articles illustrating the degree of fear that dementia can arouse. The articles portrayed a rather negative and bleak picture for those who have dementia and for those who care for them (Davies, 1995). Those working with older people who are experiencing recognized mental health needs have to work to counter these attitudes and misconceptions. There must be a realization that working with older people with mental health problems is not just a battle against illness, but against stigma, stereotype and ageism.

Professional aspects of ageism

The reader may question why a chapter titled 'Dealing with dilemmas' begins with an account of ageism and the need to reduce stigma. The answer is simple. It is the result of these attitudes and perceptions that influences not just our personal actions but also the wider population and public policies. The denial of the rights of older people may be an issue that is felt at a very personal level: the loss of choice concerning future care placement; the lack of home care services; or the destruction of personhood inside a bleak nursing home or long-stay ward.

There is also a more serious and insidious form of this loss of rights, which emanates from public and social policies. Examples of this are: the unquestioned policy on transport or lack of insight into the housing needs of older people; and the loss of index-linked state pensions or the imperceptible policy shifts that penalize older people in favour of the young. There have been the blatant episodes of ageism within the health services when age, and not need, has been the determinant of whether a service was offered or not (Thomas, 1994).

It would not be possible to discuss the dilemmas that occur without reference to the core attitudes that influence those opinions. It would be impossible to discuss risk taking without reference to our stereotypes concerning the need to protect 'vulnerable' older people. Even those of us who believe that all groups of people should have equal access and value within the health care system (and elsewhere) are tainted and influenced by those who blatantly disregard the needs of older people. Nurses are no less influenced by these inaccurate perceptions and stereotypes. Hope suggests that there are as many negative images that are sustained within nursing, as in any other area outside nursing (Hope, 1994). There is, however, a responsibility borne by those who work with older people actively to counter these negative impressions and inaccurate perceptions. Students coming into nursing need to be made aware of the value of working both with older people and with older people with mental health needs. Nurses who are in positions of influence within services, in clinical practice, management and education, need to display an enlightened attitude to working with older people in every environment. It should be a horror story of yesteryear to hear of a (nurse) manager or educationalist who suggests that a career working with older people with or without mental health needs is a 'waste of good nurses'.

Influencing carers

The issues related to the inaccurate perceptions of older people with mental health needs must also address the specific needs of carers. Carers' misconceptions can be successfully challenged, creating more positive attitudes and expectations. This is a delicate balance of education and information, founded within a strong relationship between named nurses and carers.

What, to nursing staff on a ward or in a nursing home, may appear as an older person being denied their rights, may be normal practice to a carer. A carer may insist upon the use of side rails (or cot sides) on a bed, despite the protests of the staff who may believe it is inappropriate. A carer may seek only that a residential home offers a 'safe' environment and is not concerned that staff make every effort to maximize an individual's potential through appropriate risk taking. Alternatively, a member of staff may feel unfairly treated by a carer who complains that the rights of her husband are being ignored when she discovers that he is wearing a ward cardigan when one of his own is available, or that the choice of food in the nursing home is limited. Carers' needs are becoming acknowledged as important in the complete care of any individual who has a serious mental illness. Working alongside carers creates some of the most challenging situations within nursing practice and, as a result, nurses face some very complex dilemmas.

Dealing with rights

The loss of rights for some older people can be quite staggering. Consider a completely locked ward where no-one (or very few) is detained under the Mental Health Act (Department of Health and Social Services, 1983). Although the Act may have its shortcomings, it does offer a degree of consistency and, of course, the right of appeal. A locked ward, even with the best of intentions, is a blanket form of care, which assists a minority while restraining the majority. It would appear to be a clear situation where for the 'protection' of the few, everyone is restrained.

The same may be true of a nursing home with an array of baffle locks or alarms, which aims deliberately to contain or observe people for 'their own safety'. The forms of restraint in other places may not be quite so obvious. Consider a ward or a home with rules and regulations that are so rigid and austere that they curtail activity and control residents without justification.

The main issue about such infringements of rights, which occur outside statutory powers, is that there is little or no access to an appeal structure. Older people in these situations rely upon professional staff, visitors and relatives who feel uneasy about this type of 'care' to bring about changes to practice, or to bring these concerns to the attention of managers or inspectors. This can cause problems within workplaces and is a huge dilemma for some staff. It is also a dilemma for carers who do not want to affect the ongoing care of their relative adversely. It is still unfortunately the case that, where care is available for older people with mental health problems, especially those with dementia, 'for their own good' individuals are offered a degree of supervision that most of us would feel unnecessary and heavy handed.

The balance between ensuring the safety of individuals, while maintaining their rights, appears to have swung towards overprotection. Dimond highlights the dilemma for staff when they consider the 'duty of care' expected of any individual to protect and care, especially of those involved in the welfare of others, and the basic right of the individual to freedom of movement (Dimond, 1993). She points out that to 'detain anyone without justification is actionable', and yet the absence of appropriate care is also actionable. For some carers and staff, 'appropriate care' might be the need to prevent falls at all costs, because when a fall or incident does then occur, that is viewed as negligence. Nursing staff are justifiably anxious about legal suits resulting from claims of negligence. Those caring for people who have a mental health problem are caught in a complex 'no-win situation'. If they allow free movement and a regime of care that offers maximum expression of individuality, this might result in more untoward incidents and claims of inadequate care; or, if care is regimented and denies older people their rights and individuality, this may result in the denial of choice, freedom and liberty.

There is a tightrope of choices to be walked in whichever environment one works and there are no definitive answers. Individual practitioners need to judge each situation as they find it. If the situation makes them feel 'uneasy', then there is probably an aspect of the care that needs reassessment. The degree of personal feelings of comfort or discomfort with a given set of circumstances will depend upon a host of factors, including previous experience, personal philosophy, the managerial influence, carers' perceptions, and current 'accepted' good practice. There is a trend towards more restrictive practice in all environments (perhaps as a result of the fear of litigation), which tolerates fewer risks. As a result, some nursing care has tended to err on the side of caution in relation to safety and protection, with the resultant loss of some basic rights.

The promotion of this high level of safety for older people can seriously impair wellbeing. Goodwin and Mangan (1985) have pointed out that 'the biggest risk' that older people face on entering institutional care is that they will 'suffocate under the cushion of care'. Our desire to protect older people can lead to their loss of status as individuals, and to them becoming mere objects for nursing performances and safe-keeping. Bennet and Kingston (1993) claim that these forms of structured care soon become forms of abuse.

This was graphically illustrated by an article in *The Guardian*, in which a combination of uniformity and drabness was the major theme to care (Bennet, 1994). This uniformity of care and of risk management is then reflected in the lack of individuality offered to older people with mental health needs. It amounts to a denial of rights and a lack of appropriate care. In its extreme form, it amounts to abuse.

Rights and restraint

Restraint is still viewed as a physical means of control. However, restraint is exercised in many different forms, some of which are very obvious and others which are almost unseen. In their observation of practice, Hughes and Wilkin (1989) reported the conveyer-belt like mentality to care and the description of regimented practices like 'toileting' where older people were treated as objects upon whom care was performed. This is a clear example of abuse in the form of work practices that constrain activity, limit choice and diminish the quality of life. Sometimes, the worst forms of abuse are not through the very obvious use of restraints or locked doors, but by everyday care activities that constrain and reduce freedom. The Royal College of Nursing (1992a) has outlined the major issues around restrictive care practices:

- Cot sides
- Harnesses
- Sedative drugs
- Baffle locks
- Arranging furniture to impede movement
- Inappropriate use of nightclothes during waking hours
- Chairs whose construction is designed to immobilize

This list covers comprehensively the more overt forms of restraint but does not consider some of the more subtle forms that can be used, such as removing walking aids, using slippers when shoes are available, and taking away spectacles and hearing aids. As suggested earlier, some institutions have rules and regulations that are overzealous in deliberately constraining activity and reducing choice. A loss of choice should be seen as a loss of rights and a restraint on activity.

Choice was identified by the Social Services Inspectorate as a key principle in any shared residence. This can easily be observed in various choices at meal times, including a choice from the menu, or the choice of clothes offered (Department of Health, 1989). Current society appears to pride itself on the extent of choice and political thought reverberates to notions of 'the rights of the individual'. The Patient's Charter has provided a core theme of choice and individual service (Department of Health (NHS Executive), 1992), but charters and pronouncements that suggest that everybody has the same level of choice and the same access to rights ring hollow. Bennet (1994) suggests that 'for most impoverished older people everything depends upon luck'. He suggests that services are far from consistent and that choice is only really available to a few. Older people who live in an institution have already lost their homes and their new home is unlikely to be able to offer the range of freedoms and choices that they previously enjoyed. Care offered in many nursing homes and continuing care wards is not always ideal and, if one is seeking care that offers a full range of choice and an opportunity to reach one's full potential, this is likely to be available only to those who are able to pay well for that luxury. Real choice is only for those who can afford it. Even those who live in their own homes do not have the range of choices for support that have been espoused by policy makers. As a consequence, they are restrained by the political and social circumstances in which they find themselves.

Kitwood (1993a) suggests that in the care of people with dementia, rigid regimes lead to loss of fulfilment and of personhood. An overreliance upon structure and rules reduces activity and constrains the ability to achieve maximum personhood. Kitwood uses the term personhood to describe the wholeness of an individual; he believes that people with dementia conventionally receive forms of care that constantly undermine their personhood. These destructive care practices are reflected in the interactions that occur between the carer and the person experiencing dementia. The content of these interactions creates the conditions under which individuals feel humiliated and depersonalized. Kitwood outlines several common ways in which this can occur, including:

- Treachery
- Infantilization
- Disempowerment
- Outpacing
- Objectification
- Banishment
- Intimidation

Any 'assault' on an individual's rights can lead to a loss of their personhood. Kitwood has suggested that enhanced care for people who are experiencing dementia requires a complete change in the way in which these individuals are viewed. When the above areas are accepted as activities that undermine the relationships between individuals experiencing dementia and their carers, then care will begin to improve. Kitwood believes a person with dementia needs to be seen as an individual requiring understanding and support, rather than as someone having a collection of problems that have to be solved. When this has been achieved, the degree to which an individual experiencing dementia is 'restrained' will be markedly reduced (Kitwood, 1993b).

Care settings that ignore the right to privacy in the misguided belief that everyone needs to be watched 'for their own safety', are restraining individuals' life styles. They are constraining their normal activities and denying the right to privacy (Department of Health, 1989). This may include restricted access to relatives and loved ones through overrigid visiting hours or maybe the lack of access to a telephone or letter-writing facilities. It is interesting that the revised Department of Health guidelines to the Mental Health Act explicitly discuss access to telephones for those who are detained (Department of Health and Welsh Office, 1993). Although most older people with mental health problems are not detained, good practice would be to ensure access to telephones for everyone and to encourage the facilitation of their use.

Restraint takes many guises; often the more subtle forms are the most dangerous. The overuse of cot sides may be an overt form of restraint, but it may reflect a more serious and covert institutional form of restraint, which is only evident in policies and practices away from the bedside.

Good practice is not about everyone having the same care; it is about everyone having access to the same quality of care. The RCN guidelines for good practice in relation to restraint offer sound advice and a good starting point (Royal College of Nursing, 1992). Essentially, good practice is about everyone having a thorough assessment which then leads to an individual prescription of nursing care (Crump, 1992). That plan may include the use of a cot side; it may include an explicit level of observation; it may involve the use of drugs to help to reduce overactivity during an acute phase of an illness; or it may involve reduced access to kitchens.

These 'restraining' activities can be seen as aspects of good care when individual patients have been properly assessed, planned and evaluated, and also as explicit forms of poor practice when they have been applied without thought and applied to all patients. When a care plan prescribes a form of restraint, the prescribing nurse needs to be able to justify that intervention. Given the same set of circumstances would a colleague with similar expertise and experience feel able and comfortable if prescribing the same care?

It is probably the case that where there is nursing care there will also be forms of restraint and that all nursing staff are involved in activities that restrain patients. Any intervention that is invasive, either physically or psychologically, may be viewed as potentially restraining and nurses should be aware that all their actions need to be measured and calculated. Actions that are carried out without thought may be forms of care that in themselves restrain. Given the degree of stigma, the prevalence of social and political ageism, and nursing care that is given without thought, older people with mental health problems are restrained throughout a wider set of circumstances than any other group. The first step to removing these constraints and restraints is to accept that they exist. Once they are acknowledged then the process of removing them can begin.

Risk taking

Negotiating life is a risky business. Surviving life to seventy or eighty years of age is an achievement of perseverance, and a result of good fortune and making the right decisions. Risks of all descriptions will have been faced. Some of those risks will have been taken voluntarily, but for others there will have been no choice. Risk is an everyday phenomenon and it is accepted that some people take more risks than others; however, we all take them. It is strange then, that on entering hospital, or other nursing and residential care areas, there is a sudden desire to take away all risk and create havens of safety. The reason for this safety is the perception that older people are destined to injure themselves and need protecting. This protection can lead to stifling levels of care, which become a greater hazard to health than any perceived risk in 'normal' activities (Goodwin and Maugan, 1985).

The resulting absence of normal risk in any institution is that people's lives become mundane and dull. There is a complete loss of zest for day-to-day activities (Counsel and Care, 1993a). Older people in overprotective care can be said to be in a position where they are stifled with kindness. The absence of an opportunity to take part in normal activities may be a reflection of a care environment that does not value choice or individuality. The benefits of activity and leisure are supported in a *Counsel and Care* publication on the provision of activity within care homes. One of its conclusions was that 'homes have a tendency to become isolated and unstimulating environments' (Counsel and Care, 1993b). In bleak environments where emptiness is accepted as the norm, there can be a downward spiral of increasing despondency and dependency. This 'overcare' with an emphasis on safety could be easily viewed as a blatant form of abuse. Justification stems from the notion that, because carrying out certain activities is perceived as too great a risk, it can therefore be relegated to a minor issue (Counsel and Care, 1993a).

The King's Fund produced a landmark document outlining five major principles of care in working with older people who had dementia (King's Fund, 1986):

- People with dementia have the same human value as anyone else irrespective of their degree of disability or dependence.
- People with dementia have the same varied human needs as anyone else.
- People with dementia have the same rights as other citizens.
- Every person with dementia is an individual.
- People with dementia have a right to forms of care which do not exploit family and friends.

Although these principles were written in relation to the care of people with dementia, the word 'dementia' could be dropped and the principles could be applied in a much wider context. In the discussion there is a simple statement suggesting that 'the [daily] schedule offers some of the variety of everyday life'. The simplicity of this statement belies its powerful message. If there is one thing about the lives of people with dementia and others in care, it is that they do not reflect normal everyday life: there is little excitement, there is little variation and there is almost no risk.

It is not suggested that the lives of people with mental health problems should be a roller coaster of excitement and risk; however, there is a strong case for accepting that some risk is healthy and beneficial. Counsel and Care (1993a) suggest that 'without risks, life would be impoverished'. They offer a persuasive argument for the right to take risks and present a case to show that denying people the opportunity to take any risks is unlawful. Counsel and Care encourage the practice of risk-taking activities and restraint being specifically covered in care plans. This would indicate that thought must be given to these crucial areas of care on an individual basis and that they should form part of the range of specific nursing interventions.

Attitudes towards normal activity are changing slowly, but perhaps there is one group still to convince, namely, the relatives and loved ones of those who come into care. There still exists a powerful feeling in the wider community that older people need to be protected; that relatives should have this strong feeling is therefore no surprise. They are often seeking a safe haven for their loved one and do not want anything to intrude upon that safety.

There is a multitude of feelings and emotions when a carer can no longer cope at home, especially in relation to someone with dementia (Lay and Woods, 1984). If staff are unable to grasp the need for normal activity, and the concept of the resultant normal risk which that involves, then they will not be able to pass those ideas on to relatives and carers and the cycle of accepting the status quo will continue. If relatives are not exposed to ideas of normal activity and normal risk, then they will always expect the overprotection that is the norm in many wards and residential homes. The issue then may be one of defining acceptable and normal risk and activity. This can only come as a result of building up an understanding of the previous history of the person in care and attempting to continue their level of activities and risk-taking. There will be some who took very few risks in life, who would not wish for a busy and active life; however, there will be some who were adventurous and accepted risk as the essence of living.

The concept of 'acceptable risk' is one that may take a while for a near relative or friend to understand fully. It requires a close and honest relationship between the patient, the carer and the nursing team in order to develop the trust that will result in the acceptance of normal activity and normal risk. By building up this trust and showing what can be achieved, relatives will be able once again to share in this activity and the pleasure that this can bring.

As a consequence of this process of responsible risk taking, there is increasing pressure on all professionals to ensure that its practice is not going to lead to any claims for compensation (Dimond, 1993). This may, in turn, lead to increasingly wary professionals who believe that introducing normal 'risk-laden' activity will result in the danger of disciplinary procedure. Supportive managers who believe in the need to maintain the rights of the (older) individual are therefore fundamental if staff are to feel confident about promoting a normal level of activity and a normal acceptable level of risk.

Decision making

Older people with mental health problems are often excluded from the decisions that influence their lives. Even when they are included in the decision making, their choices may be usurped by other 'more' competent younger people (Barrowclough and Fleming, 1991). This could be a decision relating to a major operation or procedure. The initial discussion about what should happen is often with the 'assumed' next of kin ignoring the fact that the older person has a right to that knowledge first. It completely ignores the concept of confidentiality and that the patient may wish to withhold this information from the assumed next of kin. It may be the case that the patient does not accept a family member as next of kin; perhaps a close next-door neighbour or home care worker has the trust and confidence of the patient. It also assumes that the older person and the next of kin share the same set of values and that the opinion of the next of kin will reflect the older person's opinions. It is as if, once in hospital, the older person loses personhood and any degree of self-determination, whatever his or her abilities (Crump, 1991).

The situation is worse still for an older person with dementia, who has even less access to the relevant information and whose competence to make decisions is assumed to be completely absent. Downie and Calman (1987) discuss the issue of the autonomous person in relation to the ability to make choices or decisions and to be able to carry out those choices. The ability to make decisions and carry them through is a mark of 'the person'. Actions that restrict an individual's ability to make decisions 'injure him as a person'. Taking away an individual's right to make decisions is removing a basic premise of autonomy and reflects an absence of respect for the individual. Downie (1989) suggests that the ability to be autonomous is not a case of all or nothing and that this relates to the relative states of competence. There will be some who are competent in decision making in one area and not competent in another because of the nature and complexity of those decisions.

A heavy responsibility for decision making is placed upon, or taken on by, other people; this is especially true of professionals. Hillan (1993) puts forward a decision-making model, which takes into account the limitations of the individual. The model is aimed at ensuring that a person can participate as fully as possible in the decision-making process. This is based upon:

- Judging where a patient's choice is constrained and where it should be free.
- Offering honest choices rather than pseudo choices
- Discovering ways to present a choice that circumvents as far as possible the obstacles imposed by illness or handicap.

This model provides a framework for maximizing the choices offered to someone who has an impaired ability to make decisions. The focus then becomes whether or not these decisions are taken into account. Norman (1987b) suggests that doctors overrule the considered opinion of some older people, particulary if they feel they are not 'lucid enough' to make the 'right' decision. It is clear that there is a conflict between the autonomy of the individual and what is seen as the best interests of that person. As long as the decision made by the older person is in line with what the professionals believe is in their best interests, then the decision is accepted. If there is any dissent, the professional could then take the option to suggest that the individual was unable to decide for himself or herself anyway, as proved by the unacceptable (to the professional) decision that was made. This could be viewed as medical paternalism, and could best be described as the assumption (by medical practitioners) that doctors know best. This has been well illustrated by Illich (1977), who describes the power and authority both vested in and accepted by medical practitioners.

However, nursing staff should not consider themselves untainted by this kind of paternalism. There are models of care that turn patients into objects and for whom everyday decisions are made. Earlier it was suggested that it was not the major issues that cause concern and dilemma, but the small (but important) everyday issues. It is nurses who have power over the minute details of an individual's day. It is nurses who may, without thinking, make decisions for people in every aspect of their lives, when in actual fact they may be perfectly able to perform those activities themselves. This arrogance shows a complete absence of thought and respect for the individuals in their care. The danger is that nursing staff will not realize that they are doing anything wrong; they will consider that they are 'acting in the best interest' of the patient. Downie (1989) considered that autonomy or the ability to make decisions is not a constant state. There may be times when it is appropriate to help patients to make decisions; however, it should not be assumed that this will be the case on a future occasion.

Good practice would be to enable every individual to make as many decisions as is possible without assistance. When decision making becomes an issue, decisions should be made *with* the individual and not *for* the individual, while offering the minimum of assistance possible. These issues are often about making judgements about an individual's ability in decision making and in making choices. That judgement should not fall upon one person but upon a team of people who know the individual well.

Advocacy

This discussion leads neatly into the concept of advocacy, which is an issue that is increasingly discussed in the nursing literature. The United Kingdom Central Council for Nursing, Midwifery and Health Visiting (1992) has highlighted the nursing role in advocacy, which they suggest is an essential skill for the professional practitioner. Hillan (1993) states that advocacy has several dimensions, including 'rights, protection, defending and pleading'. This wide range of roles may cause the nurse advocate to feel compromised and thus lead to less effective advocacy. The King's Fund (1986) suggests that there is a conflict of interest in professional advocacy. It argues that the presumption upon which this advocacy rests is a 'coincidence' of interest between users and providers. In reality, it is argued, there are irreconcilable differences between users and providers, and, if the best interests of both parties are to be served, the differences need to be accepted and understood.

Decision making and advocacy are linked themes. The King's Fund (1986) document is clear: 'If people cannot/do not participate in the decisions which affect their lives, then conflicts of interest become a growing problem'. The work of Goffman (1961) showed how an institution can become the controlling influence in people's lives. Without checks and counterbalances, there is a corrupting nature to this power and control. If one person, or group, consistently makes decisions for another party, then there is a strong possibility that the views of this party will become lost or diminished. Hobman et al. (1994) has also argued for the complete independence of advocates for older people. In situations in which important decisions need to be made, there should be strenuous efforts to provide advocates who are truly independent and free from any conflict of interest. Only then can the best interests of older persons be served.

Informed consent

A theme that is closely connected to decision making and advocacy is the issue of consent and also of informed consent. Older people who have agreed to enter hospital have given their verbal consent and thereby also agree to a range of procedures and care. Although most people do not consider that they have given explicit consent, their presence and cooperation is viewed as a form of consent. It has been argued elsewhere that there are very few people who are given all the relevant facts and information about a stay in hospital (Crump, 1991). Without that information, individuals are unable to make truly informed decisions and cannot therefore give informed consent. Indeed, it is often the most important information that is lacking, that is, the very information that might influence the decision itself. The reluctance to give information may be seen by professionals as 'acting in the best interests' of the individual represented by the simplistic belief that 'what you don't know, can't hurt you'. The arrogance in believing this is paternalism at its extreme.

The situation of consent is relatively straightforward when the individual is accepted to be 'competent'. It becomes more difficult when that competence is in doubt (Dimond, 1993). The issue of decision making and the older person with mental health problems is complex. The historical context is that large institutions and paternalistic bodies made decisions for all people, as Goffman (1961) has described. There is now an increasing need to allow everyone access to the right to make their own decisions. Where the ability to make decisions is impaired, systems need to be created and sustained to ensure the maximum level of participation in all aspects of decision making, from the small everyday issues to those that are important and complex. As Dimond (1993) points out 'no-one can give consent on behalf of the mentally incompetent adult' other than within the confines of the Mental Health Act.

It is a case of always putting the interests of the individual first, and seeing the whole picture, not just the portion in which one party is professionally involved. This calls for dialogue with other professionals and a degree of conflict in order to find the most appropriate answer. Acting in the best interests of someone else sometimes means saying things that others might find uncomfortable, but, by challenging an established view, the outcome is more likely to reflect the real interests of the patient/client and not those of any one particular group. A good test for nursing staff is to ask themselves whether other practitioners would take the same stance or approach in similar circumstances. It is suggested here that the best that can be done for older people whose competence is in question, is to offer them every opportunity to make decisions themselves before someone else steps in to do it for them.

Abuse and inadequate care

Until recently, the abuse of older people was an issue that was rarely discussed. Abuse is a sensitive subject and gives rise to uneasiness. It is often difficult to accept that abuse has happened, and therefore it is sometimes more comfortable to feign ignorance. Whether it is of children, partners or older people, there is still a tremendous resistance to acknowledging its existence fully.

The abuse of older people is not a single issue. It is not confined to just one group of people and it is not confined to one type of abuse. Bennet and Kingston (1993) suggest that part of the problem of old age abuse is its very ill-defined nature. There is also the issue of abuse through the absence of care, and the term 'inadequate care' comes to the fore.

Eastman (1994) describes abuse of older people as:

the physical, emotional or psychological abuse of an older person by a formal or informal carer. The abuse is the violation of a person's human and civil rights by a person or persons who have power over the life of a dependent.

There is no mention here of the abuse of position to take financial advantage or any aspect of the issue of time. The Royal College of Nursing Focus Working Group on Abuse (1992b) defined it as:

the ongoing inability of an informal carer to respond adequately to meet the needs of a dependent older person. This may result in the violation or loss of that person's human rights.

This tends to ignore the abuse of older people by carers within formal residential or nursing situations. It is difficult to create an exact definition of abuse that is comprehensive, yet concise. Perhaps it is easier to view the abuse of older people as any action that causes a reduction in the quality of their life. This gives the opportunity to see abuse in its widest context. However, the absence of any workable definition may lead to problems in assessment, in legal settings and in recording for research processes.

Until recently, there was a view that the abuse of older people was an issue related to a high-risk group with certain distinct characteristics. Traditionally, these were (Tomlin, 1989):

- Age over 75 years
- Female
- Roleless within the family
- Functionally impaired
- Unable to fulfil activities of daily living
- Lonely and fearful
- Living at home with, or near to, adult children

There is an uncomfortable feeling here that the consequences of abuse are the 'fault' of the abused. Although the similarities between child and old age abuse are not great, it would be outrageous to suggest that a child was responsible for being abused. In fact, this feeling of an abused child of 'being responsible' is one that is the first to be challenged. The same is true for an abused or battered partner. To blame the victim appears to be counterproductive.

Fulmer and O'Malley (1987) have suggested that there are other equally important similarities in cases of 'inadequate care'. They prefer the use of this term to describe the situation in which someone has been abused. They point to other circumstances apart from those conventionally accepted as risk factors. Their analysis adds to the understanding of the situation of abuse and inadequate care. These factors include:

- Those with chronic progressive disabling illnesses that exceed their carer's ability to cope
- Carers with a personal history of substance misuse or violent behaviour, or a family member with the same
- Carers who are financially dependent upon the person for whom they care
- Those who live in a family where there is a history of spouse or child abuse
- Those who reside in institutions that have a history of poor care
- Those whose carers suddenly have an increase in their personal stress from other sources

There is an obvious shift here away from the abused person to the abuser. Bennet and Kingston (1993) believe that the concept of the overburdened carer who is caring for a 'classic victim' needs to be seriously reviewed. There is an urgent requirement to take more account of the needs, histories and current situations of carers. This is especially in relation to mental health needs and histories of substance misuse and/or previous familial violence.

There is danger in highlighting the issue of inadequate care in the informal setting and causing abuse by paid carers in formal settings to be brushed aside. The potential for abuse within an institution may be on an individual basis or on an institutional level, with care being organized in such a way as to constitute abuse.

The process of moving care from NHS long-term care facilities to independent establishments in the community has also moved some of the institutional abuse from large asylums to smaller care settings. Although care in many nursing homes is outstanding, there are increasing numbers of reports of the abuse of older people (Easton, 1993). With a change in the main source of continuing care for older people with mental health problems, there should also be an awareness of the enormous pressure that some staff feel when caring in isolated community settings with little support or educational opportunity.

Good practice for nursing staff in identifying abuse or inadequate care is in relation to prevention and early intervention to support both the carer and the abused older person. For the over-seventy-five-year-olds there are now annual health checks; this may be a way of screening those who are in situations that are likely to stimulate abuse. Practice nurses may well be involved in the screening process and should be aware of the different aspects of abuse and the range of risk factors. Community psychiatric nurses are also well placed to monitor and detect the danger signs early.

If abuse or inadequate care is already evident, then extreme tact will need to be employed. The techniques available to uncover old age abuse/inadequate care are in their infancy compared with the techniques used to uncover child or spouse abuse. Good practice would suggest that removing the person from the abuse situation should only happen in very rare circumstances. It may be that there is scope for supportive work, offering help to both the older person and the carer. There will also be times when there is evidence of inadequate care that could be rectified with added services. There may be cases when a carer needs help from community or specialist mental health services.

There is an urgent need to raise the profile of abuse and inadequate care and make its recognition easier. Bennet and Kingston (1993) believe that there may be a three to five per cent prevalence of inadequate care reported by older people. This may prove as big an issue as other forms of abuse. Our current understanding may be the tip of the iceberg.

Conclusion

Although a particular individual's rights may be preserved there could be other individuals who find their rights have been unfairly denied or reduced. There is not always a single answer to a particular issue of individual rights.

One of the problems with discussing the dilemmas involved within the 'rights and risks' debate is that people immediately think of major philosophical issues of an academic nature. In practice, it is not the issues of life and death that cause most concern, but the everyday events that need to be resolved quickly: not the issue of physical restraint, but the degree to which the environment itself restrains; not the risks involved in allowing people to explore freely away from the clinical area, but the risks involved in allowing people to use kitchens to make tea and sandwiches; or not the opportunity to make a choice about a major operation, but the opportunity to choose the colour of clothes or food from a menu or to bathe or remain unwashed. Sometimes the larger issues can be resolved easily, but the smaller ones take on a complexity that is difficult to grasp and even more difficult to solve.

Preserving people's rights is a much more difficult task than taking them away; it takes thought, energy and perseverance. Taking them away requires only the absence of thought. The issue of rights and risks is not one where very many cases can be seen merely as 'black or white'. Mostly it is having to find a compromise between two opposing ideals, which both have their merits. With thought and application an answer will emerge, which will offer the balance between rights and risks, between choice and lack of choice and between good practice and poor.

None of us is entirely free to do exactly want we want. There are constraints placed upon our actions, freedoms and access. These are largely accepted in order to maintain a safe and stable society. On the roads, there are laws and regulations to make driving safer for everyone. In making the roads safer, there are corresponding losses in some of the individuals' right of expression. This is true of the laws concerning the wearing of crash helmets on motorbikes. There are laws governing the access to information that is of a 'sensitive' nature, which will be true of information about a nation's armed forces. There is a general acceptance that this is a necessary measure for the security of everyone. The differences in opinion that come from these 'accepted restraints' concern the extent of these constraints upon our activities, access to information and rights. Dialogue and discussion is crucial if the right balance is to be struck. This dialogue, even conflict, could be argued to be the basis of democracy. The same is true within nursing. If there is no dialogue concerning the nature of rights and risks, and choice and restraint, within nursing care, then practice will cease to move forward. Good nursing practice in relation to these issues is to be constantly aware of the dialogue and debate around such issues.

We all accept some constraints and, although these do affect our rights, this is usually felt to be an acceptable compromise and will be with our full knowledge and consent. There are times when the rights of individuals are deliberately curtailed against their wishes. A criminal or civil offence can carry with it the penalty of going to prison. The Mental Health Act has the provision to detain people without their consent (Department of Health and Social Services, 1983). Again this is within the accepted law and is perceived by most to be for the greater good. Contained within these laws and codes is the provision for appeal and a second opinion. These safety mechanisms help to ensure that it is only those who really need to have their liberty and rights curtailed who are 'restrained'.

The degree of concern over rights and liberties that is apparent in statutory powers does not seem to stretch to the care of older people with mental health problems, who are outside this system. Norman (1982) suggests that older people receive forms of care that restrict choice and are based not upon any accepted law but upon convention, perception and custom. It is accepted that entry into care can involve 'considerable sacrifices of personal freedom' (Crump, 1992). This loss of freedom and choice would be viewed as a major loss of civil rights by most people, but it is accepted as normal practice in the care of older people with mental health problems. There continues to be an acceptance that, in order to nurse or care for older people, there is also a need to protect and control them. This protection can lead to excessive amounts of regulation and observation, and an unnecessary curtailment of liberty.

The whole area of rights and risks is very complex. It always raises nurses' levels of anxiety as they search for the definitive answer. It is hoped that this chapter has raised an awareness of the issues and of the difficulties in achieving the balance between rights and risks, decision making and good practice. No two people will hold the same opinion concerning what is right and what is wrong. Often, these extremes are not useful and it is better to view 'the answer' to these complex issues as degrees towards the extremes. For us all, there will be a position between maximizing rights and taking risks where we will feel most comfortable. This understanding will not come without thought and an appreciation of all the available schools of thought. Armed with this information, everyone should find his or her own position, which, of course, is as individual as the people who find themselves in our care.

References:

Barrowclough, C. and Fleming, I. (1991). In *Ethical Issues in Mental Health*. (P. J. Barker, and S. Baldwin, eds.), pp. 68–83, London: Chapman and Hall.

Bennet, C. (1994). Ending up. *The Guardian*, Oct. 8, pp. 12–20.

Bennet, G. and Kingston, P. (1993). *Elder Abuse, Concepts, Theories and Interventions*. London: Chapman and Hall.

Brayne, C. and Ames, D. (1988). In *Mental Health and Old Age*. (B. Gearing, C. Brayne and D. Ames, eds.). pp. 27–35, Chichester: Wiley/Open University Press.

Counsel and Care. (1992). *What if they hurt themselves*. London: Counsel and Care.

Counsel and Care. (1993a). *The Right to Take Risks*. London: Counsel and Care.

Counsel and Care. (1993b). *Not Only Bingo*. London: Counsel and Care.

Crump, A. (1991). Your uninformed consent. *Nurs. Stand.* **13**(25), 44.

Crump, A. (1992). Restless spirits. *Nurs. Times*, **88**(21), 26–28.

Davies, J. (1995). Untitled series of articles. *Daily Mail*, March 22–25.

Department of Health. (1989). *Homes Are for Living In*. London: HMSO.

Department of Health. (1990). *The NHS and Community Care Act*. London: HMSO.

Department of Health. Social Services Inspectorate. (1992). *Confronting Elder Abuse*. London: HMSO.

Department of Health. Social Services Inspectorate. (1993). *Standards for the Residential Care of Elderly People with Mental Disorders*. London: HMSO.

Department of Health and Social Services. (1983). *The Mental Health Act*. London: HMSO.

Department of Health and Welsh Office. (1993). *Code of Practice*. London: HMSO.

Department of Health (NHS Executive). (1992). *The Patients' Charter*. London: HMSO.

Dimond, B. (1993). Extracting consent. *Elderly Care*, **5**(2), 14–15.

Downie, R. S. (1989). Paternalism and the rights of professionals to interfere. In *Proceedings of Age Concern Conference*, Edinburgh. Quoted in Hillan, E. M. (1993). Nursing dementing elderly people: ethical issues. *J. Adv. Nurs.*, **18**, 1889–1894.)

Downie, R.S. and Calman, K.C. (1987). *Healthy Respect*. London: Faber.

Eastman, M. (1994). *Old age abuse: a new perspective*, 2nd ed. London: Chapman and Hall.

Easton, L. (1993). Open to abuse. *Nurs. Times*, **89**(44), Bibliography:

Fulmer, T. T. and O'Malley, T. A. (1987). *Inadequate care of the elderly: a health perspective on abuse and neglect*. New York: Springer Publishing. (Quoted in G. Bennet and P. Kingston, (1993) *Elder abuse: concepts, theories and interventions*. London: Chapman Hall).

Goffman, E. (1961). *Asylums: essays on the social situation of mental patients and other inmates*. Harmondsworth; Penguin.

Goodwin, S. and Mangan, P. (1985). Cosmic nursing: solitude and sanity. *Nurs. Times*, 7 August, 45–47.

Hillan, E. M. (1993). Nursing dementing elderly people: ethical issues. *J. Adv. Nurs.*, **18**, 1889–1894.

Hobman, D., Hollingbery, R., Means, R., Lart, R. and Smith, J. (1994). *More Power to our Elders*. London: Counsel and Care.

Hope, K. W. (1994). Nurses' attitudes towards older people: a comparison between nurses working in acute medical and acute care of the elderly settings. *J. Adv. Nurs.*, **20**, 605–612.

Hughes, B. and Wilkin, D. (1989). Physical care and quality of life in residential homes. *Ageing Soc.*, **7**, 399–425.

Illich, I. (1977). *Medical Nemesis*. New York: Bantam Books

King's Fund. (1986). *Living Well Into Old Age*. London: King's Fund.

Kitwood, T. (1993a). Towards a theory of dementia care: the interpersonal process. *Ageing Soc.*, **13**, 51–67.

Kitwood, T (1993b). Discover the person not the disease. *Dementia Care*, **1**, 16–17.

Lay, C. and Woods, B. (1984). *Caring for the Person with Dementia: a Guide for Families and Other Carers*. London: Alzheimer's Disease Society.

Midwinter, E. (1988). *Out of Focus: Old Age, the Press and Broadcasting*. London: Centre for Policy on Ageing.

Norman, A. (1982). *Mental Illness in Old Age: Meeting the Challenge*. London: Centre for Policy on Ageing.

Norman, A. (1987a). *Aspects of Ageism*. London: Centre for Policy on Ageing.

Norman, A. (1987b). *Rights and Risk*. London: Centre for Policy on Ageing.

Royal College of Nursing. (1992a). *Focus on Restraint*. Harrow: Scutari Projects.

Royal College of Nursing. (1992b). *Guidelines for nurses: abuse and older people*. London: RCN.

Stokes, G. (1992). *On Being Old: the Psychology of Later Life*. London: Falmer Press.

Thomas, L. (1994). Editorial. *Elderly Care*, **6**, 3.

Tomlin, S. (1989). *Abuse of elderly people: an unnecessary and preventable problem*. London: British Geriatric Society.

United Kingdom Central Council. (1992) *Code of Professional Conduct*, London: UKCC.

Wynne-Harley, D. (1991). *Living dangerously: risk-taking, safety and older people*. London: Centre for Policy on Ageing. London.

10

Quality assurance and standard setting in hospitals

Peter Hasler and Susan Anstey

Quality assurance and the provision of mental health care to older people

Quality assurance

Quality assurance is used to make sure that the quality of a service is acceptable and will continue to be so; in other words, a process of looking at the quality of what is provided, identifying areas for improvement and taking corrective action. Oakland (1993) describes quality assurance as the prevention of quality problems through planned and systematic activities. This includes the establishment of a an effective quality management system and the assessment of its adequacy. It also includes the auditing and review of the quality system itself.

Quality assurance measurement is often expressed in terms of an adequate structure and the appropriate processes that will lead to the desired outcomes. The aim of quality assurance management is to demonstrate that continuous quality improvement mechanisms are in place.

This chapter explores some common themes of which nurses working with older people in mental health care need to be aware. It also gives some helpful pointers for those nurses who are considering setting up a local quality and audit process. The chapter starts by looking at the government reforms that have made quality assurance a central theme for all staff in the caring professions. The patient is correctly placed at the centre of the process, and nurses, who invariably spend more face-to-face time with patients than any other health professional are in a privileged position to lead many quality initiatives.

The government reforms

Reforms of the National Health Service have led to a split between those who purchase services on behalf of the local population and those who provide health services. For older people, the most noticeable impact of the reforms was the change in the provision source of funds for care in the community, which shifted from the National Health Service to Social Services. This means that a care manager now takes responsibility for funding the package of care required by an older person who is moving out of a health care into a social care situation. It has also led to a debate about the boundaries between health and social care.

The Citizen's Charter was put in place to raise the standards of public services and to respond to user requirements, as well as to give better value for money. The principles underpinning the Citizen's Charter included the setting, monitoring and publication of explicit standards. An integral part of this process must be choice and consultation with service users, to involve them in establishing these standards.

The important elements of the White paper *Working for Patients* (1989) were quality and customer responsiveness. A competitive product or a service based on a balance between quality and cost factors is the principal goal of the managed care package. Although industry has had constantly to change to survive in business, no such pressure had existed in health care until the government reforms were introduced. Developments in medical research and technology have increased the range of treatments that are available for many health needs; with this advancement has come a considerable increase in health delivery cost. Oakland (1993) described the price of quality as the continual examination of the requirements and our ability to meet them. In the light of this, a review of the health care system seems essential to look at how its finite resources can be used most effectively and to identify the priorities for health care provision.

The Patient's Charter (Department of Health, 1992) began the process of laying down a benchmark for public services. It puts the Citizen's Charter into practice by providing standards for health services. The emphasis is on the value of patients and the importance of understanding their requirements through good communication and meeting these requirements through consultation and standards setting. Since its inception in 1992, *The Patient's Charter* has increased the public's expectation for a better health service. In addition, Social Services now have a Community Charter requiring explicit standards for community care.

Setting standards and measuring satisfaction

The Patient's Charter provides a useful starting point when considering health care service delivery standards. Standard setting needs to address the areas critical to the delivery of the patient's care. These may be identified through known problems identified through complaints, incidents and accidents and the consequences of communication breakdown. Standards may need to be agreed in line with government policies and contracts from health service commissioners. Basic values underpinning the care of older people can be described broadly as those of privacy, dignity, choice, respect and independence. An agreement on critical indicators for quality will enable the cost of monitoring to be kept within the resources available. Whatever is the starting point for setting standards, one aspect is essential: standards must be real and important indicators of quality. To be truly meaningful, patients must be involved in the process of standard setting to achieve a shared understanding of the service requirements.

Developing and agreeing standards

The local strategy for standard setting and audit will determine the method of those setting standards. There are many models that nurses can use for standard setting. Donabedian (1966) provided three defined categories of structure, process and outcome, by which to measure the quality of health care. Structure describes the resources (financial, environmental, knowledge and skills) required to achieve a standard. It refers to the social and physical environment required. This can include the staffing skills, numbers and mix required. It can also refer to the equipment and buildings required. Process describes the level of activity (assessment, planning, implementation and evaluation) required to achieve the desired result. It looks at the events throughout the treatment episode, for example, the care provided from the point of referral to assessment and treatment. Outcome describes exactly what result is to be achieved, in a specific and measurable form, from the patient's or recipient's perspective. It refers to the results of the treatment package and the extent to which the patient has been helped and his or her problem resolved.

A standard statement must describe the overall level of performance of the standard. It incorporates the desired outcome and level of service or quality that can be expected. Outcome is the area that is the most difficult to measure in the care of older people. This is discussed by Green (1992) in a report on the process of care and related outcomes in the care of older people. She highlights the problems involved when patients are unable to give their view or express their satisfaction. It is argued that outcomes that demonstrate improvement in the quality of life can be more relevant than those that offer a change in health status in the care of people with a progressive illness.

The standard-setting cycle to achieve quality assurance is a continual process. The first step is to set a standard which is realistic, understandable, measurable, beneficial and achievable (known as RUMBA). The standards must be valued by those who implement them because quality is based on value judgements that must be owned and made real.

The agreed standard must be audited to measure conformance with the criteria. This leads to a plan to change and improve the process to meet or raise the standard, leading to a cycle of continuous quality improvement. Within the process, it is essential for every member of the team to realize his or her unique contribution and responsibility for maintaining and raising the quality of the input. When all team members are able to do this, it realizes the strength of the team and leads to excellence in service delivery and subsequent outcome.

Once standards are agreed there is a tendency to monitor everything, all the time. Many organizations have increased the number of administration staff to keep up with the quantity of monitoring and data collection. This has an impact on services delivered to patients as staff find themselves spending more time monitoring than delivering care. Monitoring requirements for standards must be maintained within the resources that the service has available. When there are problems with a particular aspect of service delivery, standards can be rigorously monitored and action taken towards improvement to achieve the standard. When the standards are achieved consistently, monitoring can be reduced to a few critical indicators. However, standard setting alone will not assure quality. A press report on one hospital described how it had been found that the furniture in the day room was totally unacceptable for elderly patients; the emergency call system was sometimes out of easy reach; the supply of sheets was frequently nonexistent; and there were also problems with food presentation and inappropriate cutlery. However, the response to this from the hospital spokesperson was to say that, at the last audit, the hospital had been ninety-five per cent up to standard.

This example shows the importance of agreeing the aspects of care that are valued by patients, professionals and managers. *The Patient's Charter* 'soft standards', which include respect for privacy and dignity, and respect for religious and cultural beliefs, are a helpful starting point when developing agreed standards locally.

Having agreed the standard, it is then necessary to monitor whether this is being maintained. This is commonly done through some form of audit process which may involve the staff, the patient's carers, the patient or an outside person. It is common for organizations such as the Community Health Council to undertake or be involved in this role. The process may be formal or informal, depending on the area of the audit and who requires the audit. In most health service contracts, the commissioners request formal feedback as part of their own contract-monitoring process.

The complaints procedure is another commonly used indicator of satisfaction. In order for this to be effective, it is essential that complaints are recorded. The recipients of services for older people with mental health problems tend not to complain and, often, the relatives are so grateful for any support they receive that they have to be extremely dissatisfied before a complaint is made. Even then, complaints are most commonly about the loss of property and clothing, rather than the quality of care.

Generally, it is understood that even the best services will receive complaints, and many services will encourage the process. A good complaints system can be a very effective way of receiving direct feedback and taking corrective action where necessary.

The benefits of good quality are that patients, staff and customers are satisfied; the desired outcomes are achieved; and the requirements of patients and staff are met with adequate resources; the service is reliable, and is delivered correctly and at the first attempt; and there is a good reputation for high quality information and standards.

Ovretveit (1992) provides a three-dimensional approach to health service quality:

1. Patient quality: what the patient and carers want from the service
2. Professional quality: whether the service meets needs as defined by professional providers and referers, and whether it carries out correctly the techniques and procedures that are believed to be necessary to meet patients' needs
3. Management quality: the most effective and productive use of resources within limits and directives set by higher authorities/purchasers

Quality for clients

Maxwell (1984) describes six dimensions of quality:

1. Appropriateness: the service/procedure is what the population or individual really needs
2. Equity: a fair share for all the population
3. Accessibility: services are not compromised by undue limits of time or distance
4. Effectiveness: achieving the intended benefit for the individual and for the population

5. Acceptability: services are provided such as to satisfy the reasonable expectations of patients, providers and the community

6. Efficiency: resources are not wasted on one service to the detriment of another.

Patients' views can, on occasions, be difficult to obtain. Some people do not wish to talk about their experiences; others may be unable to express themselves due to their mental health or physical problems. It is also common to find that some older people have a very low expectation of health care. After an episode of ill health, people often wish to distance themselves from any links with mental health services when they no longer require them. However, patient dissatisfaction issues are well documented (Brandon, 1981; McIver, 1991); these include the attitudes of staff and professional carers who tend to assume that people with mental illness are unable to make any valid judgements about their care. However, even in the presence of severe illness, people can express opinions about the quality of care they receive. Hannson et al. (1993) states that patients most commonly complain about the attitudes of staff and feelings of disempowerment. As Brandon (1981) points out, in psychiatry, patients are seen as a group of people who use services in a passive way and therefore complaints are infrequent.

Chui (1994) described nine quality components that were important to those who use health services:

1. The level of service provided
2. Facilities
3. Arrangements for appointment, admission and discharge
4. Access to services
5. Acceptable treatment and care
6. Relief of symptoms and improvement in quality of life
7. Treating patients with dignity
8. Involvement of patients
9. Communication between professional staff and patients

These components can be used to form the basis of a comprehensive quality cycle that will address the issues most commonly seen as important to patients.

Traditionally, health service consumers receive what those responsible for providing the service think is best. In moving towards a market-orientated organization, care providers such as NHS trusts need to find out what consumers want. Hansson et al. (1993) found that patients most valued the qualities of: caring; being interested and understanding; having respect for patients; devoting time to patients; and creating a safe treatment environment. It can be seen from the work by Hansson et al. (1993) that the nurse–patient relationship and patient information are very important aspects of patient satisfaction. Therefore, an approach towards exploring these areas is needed to empower patients.

Patients may need to be empowered to ensure that their views are heard. An independent advocacy scheme is the most common way of achieving this. Patients can also be empowered by ensuring that their views are communicated directly to the organization. This can be achieved by trust board members meeting directly with users, to hear their views without the involvement or presence of staff. Nonexecutive directors may be particularly helpful in this role.

Health providers are increasingly promoting the role of patients' representatives to complement the existing patient consultation approaches. Other approaches include focus groups, meetings, suggestion schemes and complaints systems. The role of a patients' representative aims to bridge the gap between staff and patients, which may exist because of professional relationships. The representative is in a position to collect information that will inform providers and commissioners of the areas of service development that are required in the future.

To provide a quality service, an organization is required to improve services for patients. This must be demonstrated by clinical outcomes, patients' perceptions of the services, and value for money. An organization also needs to ensure that there is continuous improvement in standards of care and services. To maintain a continuous improvement in quality the following must occur:

- Establish comprehensive agreed and measurable standards covering major aspects of care
- Monitor to ensure that performance conforms to these standards
- Audit positive and negative outcomes of care through an effective, clear and 'owned' audit process.

Professional quality

Professional quality is about considering the outcome and processes of a professional's work, using methods and techniques to measure the effectiveness and applying the results to practice. To achieve professional quality, the provider requires staff who are knowledgeable and skilled in the range of techniques necessary to assess and treat the type of patient served. Professional procedures and policies must be in place to assure practice standards and there must be a system for supervision or colleague support to give guidance.

Shaw (1986) makes the point that what constitutes good health care needs to be described so that it can be measured and improvement made. While this can be difficult to do, it is important that expectations are clearly stated. During this process, professionals often find that they are not doing what they thought they were doing. Williamson (1991) provides us with this thought on quality care: 'Offering quality care means that we will do for the patient what we are reasonably certain is necessary. There is no point in doing less and there is danger in doing more'.

Professional quality standards should be developed and integrated with patient and management quality standards in a quality management cycle (Ovretveit, 1992).

Management quality

The key to improving an organization is to address quality systematically and scientifically, in order to help staff to improve the way in which they work. Management quality is described by Ovretveit (1992) as the most efficient and productive use of resources, within limits and directives set by higher authorities/purchasers. Management quality refers to the design of processes to deliver a productive, cost-effective service through good management and to obtain the best from limited resources. Exercises to save money need to be considered carefully for 'knock on' effects. For example, holding vacant posts will increase the pressure on those who remain to deliver the accepted level of service. It often follows that there is an increase in staff sickness and absenteeism among the team and this may escalate, leading to an increase in staff turnover, which causes further disruption and low morale for those who remain. This example of cost saving may well result in increased costs longer term, affecting patient and professional quality.

The level of management quality will determine the number of mistakes made and complaints received about poor information, communication and process breakdown. When management quality is good, staff spend less time dealing with problems that are created within the service and have more time to deal with patient needs. Everyone is satisfied with the service and there is the added value of motivated staff.

In order to manage quality problems in order to take corrective action, it must be possible to identify at what point things go wrong and the amount of time wasted. Ovretveit's quality correction cycle provides a useful approach to this.

How professional and practice development can enhance patient care and quality of service provision

The care programme approach (CPA) was introduced in April 1991 and aimed to provide a network of care in the community for mentally ill people. It was hoped to achieve this by ensuring effective multidisciplinary and multiagency coordination for all patients being discharged from hospital and all those accepted by the specialist mental health services. While all such service users are provided for under CPA, the guidance suggests that three groups in particular should be considered for more extensive input:

- People with a severe mental illness with complex health and social care needs who require care management in addition to the CPA
- People with severe mental illness who require multidisciplinary care but not care management
- People accepted by the specialist mental health services who require assessment and treatment by one professional

In the care of older people with mental health needs, identifying who should be the lead agent is not always clear and has the potential to cause confusion among those who are seeking these services. Many successful services are provided jointly, and are reported to meet user needs. The care manager is an integral part of the health care multiprofessional team. A development on this theme has been the ever-increasing examples of shared care management, where either health or social services staff within a joint care management team, undertake the care management role. This model can clarify the 'grey areas' between care management and the care programme approach, and remove the repetitious assessments to which so many service users have been subjected. Joint protocols must be agreed between health and social services for the care programme approach to be delivered as a seamless service for the patient.

Another approach is to look at outcomes of health care, examining the long-term results of the care provided. When Donabedian (1966) looked at outcomes among patients several years after their treatment, he had to consider what had led to a particular outcome. He looked at aspects of the processes of treatment and care that occurred or were planned around the patient, and the structure on which the processes were based. It is a complex issue to identify all those factors that have helped or hindered a patient's progress during the course of an illness and its treatment. It is further complicated by trying to control these factors. This is particularly true in illnesses related to mental health, in which the social environment and the patient's experience have a great impact on mental wellbeing.

The NHS Executive (1996) suggests that multiprofessional clinical audit should be developed within a culture of constant evaluation of clinical effectiveness focusing on patients' outcomes. Standard setting is the responsibility of everyone in an organization. Services are rarely provided by one profession; therefore all those who contribute to individual care programmes need to be involved in the standard-setting process.

There are two approaches to assuring quality. The first is through quality performance standards; the second is by means of a quality system. These approaches are often taken separately, although it is possible to combine them. A quality system ensures that standards are set and monitored, that action is taken and evaluated, and the whole process is documented. Specifications and standards are an essential part of a quality system. Quality programmes increasingly need to detect and prevent circumstances that could lead to the occurrence of events that could cause injury or harm to a patient, employee or visitor.

The Health Advisory Service (HAS) monitors facilities for elderly and mentally ill people. It was the revelation in 1969 about poor quality care in psychiatry and mental handicap hospitals that led to the establishment of the HAS and the National Development Team for Mentally Handicapped People, which monitors institutions for people with learning disabilities. The HAS and other advisory agencies do not have established standards for assessment, but operate a peer review using a retrospective approach to health service quality. In mental health services, one approach used to establish the quality of the service is QUARTZ, a quality assessment tool for use in mental health services. This employs observational techniques and team work. It is flexible enough to be applied to different settings and types of service delivery. The QUARTZ system comprises a number of schedules covering different aspects of service quality. It has been shown to be reliable and valid.

Conclusion

Nurses, as professional practitioners, are personally accountable for their actions and standards of practice. They also, through the United Kingdom Central Council for Nursing, Midwifery and Health Visiting *Code of Professional Conduct* (1992) have a responsibility to: 'safeguard and promote the interests of individual patients and clients; serve the interests of society; justify public trust and confidence; uphold and enhance the good standing and reputation of the profession.'

The pressures of the daily workload can soon find nurses not giving to quality assurance the time and importance that it deserves. However, nurses clearly have a responsibility as individuals and as part of the wider multi-disciplinary team to treat quality seriously. Standard setting does not need to be complicated or time consuming. *The Patient's Charter* can be used as a starting point and, with patient involvement, simple but meaningful and valued standards can become part of every work area.

References

Brandon, D. (1981). *Voices of Experience. Consumer Perspectives of Psychiatric Treatment.* London: MIND.

Chui, D. (1994). Quality components in the customer – orientated health care system. *Quality World*, (May), **20**(5), 302–306.

Department of Health. (1992). *The Patient's Charter*. London: HMSO.

Donabedian, A. (1966). Evaluating the quality of medical care. *Milbank Memorial Fund Q.*, **41**, 166–206.

Government White Paper. (1989). *Working for Patients*. London: HMSO.

Green, S. (1992). Outcome measures for the elderly: a contradiction in terms. *Int. J. Health Care Quality Assurance*, **5**(4), 17–22.

Hansson, L., Bjorkman, T. and Berglund, I. (1993). What is important in psychiatric inpatient care? Quality from the patient's perspective. *Quality Assurance Health Care*, **5**(1), 41–47.

Maxwell, R. J. (1984) Quality assessment in health. *B.M.J.*, **288**, 1470–1472.

McIver, S. (1991). Obtaining the Views of Patients of Mental Health Services. London: King's Fund.

McIver, S. (1994). *Establishing Patients' Representatives*: National Association of Health Authorities and Trusts.

NHS Executive (1996) *Promoting Clinical Effectiveness: A framework for action in and through the NHS*. London: Department of Health.

Oakland, J. S (1993). *Total Quality Management: The Route to Improving Performance*. Oxford: Butterworth-Heinmann.

Ovretveit, J. (1992). *Health Service Quality: An Introduction to Quality Methods for Health Services*: Oxford: Blackwell Scientific.

Shaw, C. (1986). Introducing Quality Assurance. (King's Fund project paper). London: King's Fund.

Williamson, J. (1991) *Providing Quality Care Health Service Management*, February.

Index